Queer Interventions in Biomedicine and Public Health

AF173652

Rebecca Garden · William J. Spurlin
Editors

Queer Interventions in Biomedicine and Public Health

Second Edition

Previously published in *Journal of Medical Humanities* Volume 40, Issue 1, March 2019

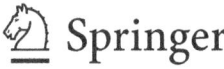 Springer

Editors
Rebecca Garden
SUNY Upstate Medical University
Syracuse, NY, USA

William J. Spurlin
Department of Arts and Humanities
Brunel University London
Uxbridge, UK

ISBN 978-3-031-29676-5   ISBN 978-3-031-29677-2   (eBook)
https://doi.org/10.1007/978-3-031-29677-2

This Springer imprint is published by the registered company Springer Nature Switzerland AG
The registered company address is: Gewerbestrasse 11, 6330 Cham, Switzerland

Contents

Journal of Medical Humanities (2019) 40:1–5
https://doi.org/10.1007/s10912-018-9533-1

Critical Healing: Queering Diagnosis and Public Health through the Health Humanities

Rebecca Garden[1]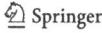

Published online: 9 August 2018
© Springer Science+Business Media, LLC, part of Springer Nature 2018

Abstract

This introduction provides an overview to a special issue on Critical Healing, which draws on queer theory, disability studies, postcolonial theory, and literary studies to theorize productive engagements between the clinical and cultural aspects of biomedical knowledge and practice. The essays in this issue historicize and theorize diagnosis, particularly diagnosis that impacts trans health and sexuality, homosexuality, and HIV/AIDS transmission. The essays also address racialization, disability, and colonialism through discussions of fiction, film, theoretical memoir, and comics, as well as biomedical discourse and knowledge.

Keywords Health humanities · Diagnosis · Transgender · HIV/AIDS · Graphic medicine · Disability · Race

The work that is done in the health humanities—at the nexus of disciplines such as literary studies, queer theory, disability studies, postcolonial theory, and medicine—investigates and exposes the social forces that have harmed, suppressed, or even eradicated those people whom medicine has defined as deviant, pathological, or disordered. Medicine and public health can benefit significantly from health humanities interventions that focus on the theory and practice of diagnosis, a phenomenon that is as capable of harm as it is of healing. According to the poet and essayist Eli Clare, diagnosis "wields immense power. It can provide us access to vital medical technology or shame us, reveal a path toward less pain or get us locked up. It opens doors and slams them shut. It holds history and creates baselines….It unleashes political and cultural forces….Diagnosis is a tool rather than a fact, an action rather than a state of being, one story among many" (2017, 41 and 45). Clare identifies the discursive and narrative dimensions of diagnosis, demonstrating how to open it up to alternative modes of knowing and to critical healing.

Critical healing, as illustrated by the essays in this special issue, is an alternative means of diagnosis and cure. It resists reductive medical narratives by excavating the possibilities of

✉ Rebecca Garden
  gardenr@upstate.edu

[1] SUNY Upstate Medical University, 618 Irving Ave., Syracuse, NY 13210, USA

meaning and by restoring the potential for multiplicities of story, particularly the narratives of bodily and psychic difference generated by those who seek healthcare. Critical healing provides the cultural tools needed for self-advocacy and self-determination. It rejects the sharp boundaries of diagnosis, which can be confining and painful when they fail to extend beyond biomedical explanations. Challenging the norms and restrictive categories that define exclusive territories of normalcy and health, critical healing recognizes the deep knowledge, authority, and ability to heal that resides in those historically marked by medicine with labels such as *disordered*, *diseased*, and *deviant*. The field of health humanities offers medicine an opportunity to engage with critical and cultural healing, to comprehend the cultural scripts, counternarratives, and performances that have strengthened individuals and communities and healed wounds caused by biomedicine itself. Critical healing contends with norms and standards that confine, exclude, and erase. It does so through modes of analysis that recognize difference and diversity and through an education in the histories and technologies of oppression. Critical healing creates space in the margins for alternatives to normalcy and health, spaces where those deemed misfits are able to flourish. Rosemarie Garland-Thomson theorizes *misfitting* as the "disjunctures that occur in the interactive dynamism of becoming" in a world that is both material and constructed by discourse (2011, 594). Misfitting creates an outcast status that occurs when there is a "discrepancy between body and world, between that which is expected and that which is," leading to injustice and discrimination through the materiality of the world as well as through social attitudes and representational practices (593). Critical healing identifies the mechanisms of that injustice and discrimination, the cultural and social forces that work through what is perceived as objective scientific knowledge, diagnosis, and treatment.

The essays in this special issue explore the social meanings and norms related to race and ethnicity, ability, class, gender, and sexuality that biomedicine generates and perpetuates through its theories and practices. While the health humanities have in the past focused primarily on the individual experiences of illness, they have not always or consistently explored the differences and variations related to these social categories. By challenging medicine's contribution to restrictive notions of fitness, the health humanities can more deeply comprehend misfitting and thus particularity, "those singularities [that] emerge and gain definition only through their unstable disjunctive encounter with an environment" (Garland-Thomson 2011, 595). Medicine's ability to heal or to harm depends on its practitioners' awareness of particularity, the singularities that can break down the boundaries between the so-called normal and pathological. Medicine must recognize those identities that have been obscured or segregated by conventional norms and diagnoses. Health humanities practices—such as critical healing—that engage with unrecognized and underrepresented identities can help make legible to medical practitioners the meanings and narratives bound up in those subjectivities and thus enable agency and strategies of resistance to diagnoses and treatments that may be harmful to particular groups or individuals.

The first essay in this special issue provides the fundamental tools for critical healing. In his essay, "Queer Theory and Biomedical Practice: The Biomedicalization of Sexuality/The Cultural Politics of Biomedicine," William Spurlin analyzes the relationship of medical knowledge and social norms, particularly in relation to biomedicine's impact on the politics of gender, sexuality, and HIV/AIDS. He also looks at how racial bias in biomedicine and social health policies have shaped access to treatment and prevention programs for HIV/AIDS in Africa. His essay investigates the intimate relations among biomedicine, culture, and society, exploring the historical links between biomedicine and nationalism by comparing U.S.

American psychiatry's characterizations of homosexuality as psychopathology with Nazi medicine's racialization of health and by identifying links to postcolonial nationalisms. Spurlin's essay reviews Michel Foucault's historicization of medical authority that assigns meaning to symptoms and has established and enforced moral and psychological as well as physical norms. His essay provides a broad historical and theoretical frame that lays the groundwork for the essays to follow.

Queer theory is Spurlin's analytical lens and mode of political engagement, enabling him to interrogate the history and politics of diagnosis and clinical practice related to gender and sexuality, examining how ostensibly objective scientific studies, diagnoses, and public health discourses have enforced gender norms and social mores and pathologized homosexuality. His essay also examines colonial medicine's sexualization and pathologization of Africanness and the way that colonial medical knowledge and practice has shaped understandings of sexuality and care for people with HIV/AIDS in postcolonial Africa today. By examining society's perceptions of deviance and immorality in people with HIV/AIDS, Spurlin identifies how both Western and heteronormative bias in public health organizations like the World Health Organization led to a critical failure to address HIV transmission in Africa and to understand how it relates to the violence and infection that are enabled by heteronormativity and homophobia. Finally, Spurlin identifies the lack of attention paid to sexuality in some of the recent work being done on structural competency and the social determinants of health. The questions at the heart of Spurlin's essay frame the critical engagements of this special issue: "How does western biomedicine continue to play a significant political role in the cultural management of gender and sexual norms? How might the relationship between the clinical and cultural spheres be better engaged in biomedical knowledge and practice, especially around the topic of sexual health, given its historic failure to recognize the impact of heteronormative assumptions…?"

Marty Fink picks up this charge to explore and theorize the relationship between biomedicine and culture with the essay "Choir Boy: Trans Vocal Performance and the De-pathologization of Transition." Fink's essay analyzes and resists the medicalization of trans identity and experience through its investigation of trans counter-fictions and cultural scripts. The essay outlines the history of the development of a clinical diagnosis of transsexuality that has created gated access to gender-confirming surgery and treatment, as well as access to employment, housing, and social services. Trans patient advocates and activists and trans theorists have identified the ways in which the medical narrative reflects the trans community's complexity and difference and how medical narrative functions as gatekeeping and can be used reductively by some clinicians. The trans community has mastered the prescribed narrative of the diagnoses of Gender Identity Disorder and Gender Dysphoria in order to access medical care. However, the medical narrative involves attesting that one was born with the "wrong body," and the diagnosis depends on expressions of hatred of one's own body, a script that has a profound impact on self-regard and self-expression. Fink's essay calls attention to the way that trans counternarratives and cultural scripts re-write the medical narrative to create greater self-determination and self-directed medical access. The trans novel Charlie Anders' *Choir Boy* describes the protagonist's refusal of gender identity in favor of an identity determined by vocal performance. It talks back to historical biomedical practices and their effects by emphasizing the "right voice" (a prepubescent treble singing voice) over the "wrong body" in its counternarrative. Fink's essay draws in part on disability studies theory, which recognizes the authority of people with embodied difference and foregrounds self-advocacy and self-determination in medical care. It looks at transition narratives in which vocal performance, rather than gender conformity, is what is most valuable.

Jordana Greenblatt's essay "The Banality of Anal: Safer Sexual Erotics in the Gay Men's Health Crisis' *Safer Sex Comix* and Ex Aequo's *Alex et la vie d'après*" analyzes the nuances of safer sex narratives in HIV/AIDS harm reduction comics to tease out the potential epidemiological effects of representations of sex. Greenblatt compares two campaigns of sexually explicit safer sex comics, one from the midst of the AIDS crisis in the mid 1980s and the other more recent. She charts how a diversity of sexual acts and sexual narratives in the earlier comics is reduced by heteronormative conventions to a singular notion of sex in the later comics, a reduction that eliminates a range of erotic experience that is less epidemiologically risky because it involves a variety of low-risk sex practices. Greenblatt's essay explores questions that are fundamental to the health humanities, such as the effects of diagnosis on the self and sexuality. It looks at the ways that health-driven narratives shape erotic experience and influence health outcomes with their scripts, especially considering what is lost when heteronormative scripts dominate. It investigates the workings and the impact of representation by looking at how one comics campaign represents a wide range of safer sex acts as highly eroticized and another restricts representations of sex and the conception of an erotic seropositive body. Greenblatt assesses the relationship between explicit and graphic representations of sex between men in these public health comics and their impact on identity, subjectivity, sexuality, and health post-diagnosis and explores the precise discursive mechanisms of representations of safer sex. Given Greenblatt's analysis, how can future public health comics validate seropositive embodiment and identity and validate safer sexual practices?

Reckoning with the power of diagnosis, Stephanie Hsu's essay "Fanon and the New Paraphilias: Towards a Trans of Color Critique of the *DSM-V*" brings the humanities to bear on biomedicine in order to look critically at the *Diagnostic and Statistical Manual of Mental Disorders,* 5th edition (or *DSM-V*), focusing on the historical tendency of the *DSM* to isolate mental health from its cultural, socio-economic, and political contexts. The essay brings Frantz Fanon's anti-racist and anti-colonial writings to bear on diagnoses related to transsexuality in the *DSM-V*. It examines the neocolonial dimensions of an earlier edition's diagnosis of Gender Identity Disorder as a gateway to access medical treatment related to gender transition, as well as access to trans-appropriate medical care. Hsu identifies the positive development in diagnoses from the *DSM-IV* to the *DSM-V*, as focus shifts from pathologizing gender identity through the earlier diagnostic category of Gender Identity Disorder to emphasizing impairment with Gender Dysphoria, given the gap or mismatch those who identify as transgendered often experience between the assigned and experienced genders. She also explores how, despite this advance, the theory behind the diagnosis nonetheless reinforces heteronormativity. Describing the difference between the narratives that trans people must tell about themselves in order to receive treatments and the reality of their varied experiences, Hsu charts how this diagnostic requirement reinforces the power imbalance between trans people and clinicians and researchers. By looking into a compelling narrative moment in Frantz Fanon's 1957 *Black Skin, White Masks*, Hsu explores Fanon's account of the psychotic nature of racism and colonialism to identify what is missing from the *DSM*'s account of trans experience: the social, political, and material contexts of mental health and embodiment. Hsu's reading also reveals how the mechanisms of the ideology of racism might shape the logic at work in the *DSM-V* diagnoses. The essay analyzes the potential costs of a diagnosis that expands access to medical care for trans people.

All of the essays in this special issue grapple with what is lost and what is gained through diagnosis and other medical narratives and modes of knowledge and authority. The essays guide our understanding and use of tools such as diagnosis and offer a means to avoid harm and work toward critical healing through a deeper knowledge of the cultural, social, political, and historical forces that shape diagnosis and shape the lived experience of embodied difference. Proposing critical engagements and counternarratives as methods of healing, these essays generate new possibilities and new models for care. This special issue theorizes and maps deeper engagements of the clinical and cultural intersections that inscribe biomedical knowledge and practice.

Acknowledgements The co-editors would like to express their heartfelt thanks to Lauren Zahn for her editorial assistance and to our anonymous peer reviewers for their excellent suggestions and insightful comments on the essays. This project began as a Medical Humanities panel at the Modern Language Association and as seminar on queer theory and biomedicine at the American Comparative Literature Association, and we are grateful to the Division on Science and Literature (MLA) and the Comparative Gender Studies Committee (ACLA) for germinating this special issue.

References

Clare, Eli. 2017. *Brilliant Imperfection: Grappling with Cure*. Durham: Duke University Press.
Garland-Thomson, Rosemarie. 2011. "Misfits: A Feminist Materialist Disability Concept." *Hypatia* 26 (3): 591-609.

J Med Humanit (2019) 40:7–20
https://doi.org/10.1007/s10912-018-9526-0

Queer Theory and Biomedical Practice:
The Biomedicalization of Sexuality/The Cultural Politics
of Biomedicine

William J. Spurlin[1]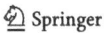

Published online: 3 August 2018

Abstract This article works across multiple disciplinary boundaries, especially queer theory, to examine critically the controversial, and often socially controlling, role of biomedical knowledge and interventions in the realm of human sexuality. It will attempt to situate scientific/medical discourses on sexuality historically, socially, and culturally in order to expose the ways in which "proper" sexual health in medical research and clinical practice has been conflated with prevailing social norms at particular historical junctures in the 20th and 21st centuries. How might the relationship between clinical and cultural spheres be better engaged in biomedical knowledge and clinical practice in understanding sexual health, given the impact of homophobic and transphobic assumptions in the diagnostic histories of homosexuality and Gender Identity Disorder in Childhood, a new diagnostic category introduced into the *DSM* following the removal of homosexuality from the *DSM-III*? The article will argue further that biomedical knowledge is always already mediated through culture by analyzing normative racial, gender, class, and sexual ideologies that regulated early understandings of the epidemiology of the HIV/AIDS pandemic in the West and in the postcolonial world while informing global health policy on HIV/AIDS. The article concludes by examining the implications of medical education for both LGBTQI patients and medical professionals, for understanding gender and sexual rights as human rights, and for thinking about new kinds of interventions, contestations, and struggles to resist continued homophobic and transphobic assumptions in biomedical practice today and their ongoing effects in the everyday world.

✉ William J. Spurlin
William.Spurlin@brunel.ac.uk

[1] Department of Arts and Humanities, Brunel University London, Uxbridge, England UB8 3PH, UK

Keywords Biomedical knowledge · Queer theory · Sexual health · Homosexuality · Gender identity disorder · Gender dysphoria · HIV/AIDS

One of the most politically contested axes of social subjectivity in contemporary culture is that of sexuality. While analyses of sexuality in biomedicine and in the humanities have, for the most part, developed along separate trajectories for different purposes, this article works across multiple disciplinary boundaries such as medical history, global and social health policy, postcolonial studies, and queer studies, as a way of examining critically the controversial, and often socially controlling, role of biomedical knowledge and interventions in the realm of human sexuality. In his book *The Birth of the Clinic*, Michel Foucault speaks of a significant discursive shift in biomedical knowledge around the end of the eighteenth century centered around "a new 'carving up' of things and the principle of their verbalization" through the process of the medical commentary (1973, xviii), which implied a new relationship between the *perceptible* and the *stateable*, between what is seen and what is said, thereby instantiating a redistribution of the relation between signifier and signified, that is, "between the symptoms that signify and the disease that is signified" (xviii-xix). In other words, according to Foucault, the medical commentary assumes an excess of the signified over the signifier, a residue of thought that has not yet been articulated in language so that the act of commenting is thought to give voice to that which has not yet been explicitly stated and is thus allowed to speak—that is, it uncovers deeper meanings by stating what has been said while simultaneously (re)stating what has not been specifically said, but has been signified (xvi). The discursive shift from the totality of the visible to the overall structure of the expressible is what occurs in the medical commentary; as Foucault more succinctly argues, "the clinical gaze has the paradoxical ability to *hear a language* as soon as it *perceives a spectacle*" (108). The mediation of the medical commentary is thought to strengthen the bond, suture the gap, between signifier and signified, between a symptom and its meaning, and give biomedicine a new discursive structure and a veneer of scientific precision, but the clinical gaze of which Foucault speaks is not without its concomitant social and cultural interpretations of the symptoms and signs of illness and disease.

Not only was there a shift in the discursive structures of western biomedicine at the end of the eighteenth century, there was a simultaneous epistemological shift in biomedical practices to the extent that medicine became linked to the destinies of nation-states. According to Foucault, this meant that medicine was no longer confined to a body of knowledge and techniques for curing ills nor concerned with the qualities of vigor, suppleness, and fluidity that were lost in illness which medical practice could restore, but biomedicine assumed a normative posture and became authorized to dictate the standards for the physical and moral relations of the individual and the broader social world in which he or she lived. As Foucault theorizes, since the nineteenth century, medicine "was regulated more in accordance with normality than with health"; that is to say, in considering the life of groups or societies, the life of the race, as well as psychic life later in the century, biomedical concepts became structured around the polarity of the normal and the pathological (34-35). Interestingly, it is also at the end of the eighteenth century, according to George Mosse, that the rise and proliferation of modern nationalisms in Europe were linked to middle class norms of the body and sexuality (Parker, Russo et al. 1992, 2), thus instantiating a link between the moral and physical (and later psychological) health of the individual and the health of the state—and the conflation of good health with social conformity.

The legacy of these two historical shifts articulated by Foucault, as well as the fusion of the medical and juridical spheres, which often forms the basis for citizenship, rights, and national belonging, are especially important since biomedical knowledge, and its concomitant social authority on sexuality, not without its political biases, had, from the nineteenth century, not only influenced and buttressed colonial power and rising fascist movements in Europe in the early twentieth century, but also, in the aftermath of imperialism, formed the basis for directing social health policies within western contexts and in the postcolonial and developing world. Coincidentally, it is within the context of biomedical and psychiatric discourses in the mid-nineteenth century that homosexuality, as a form of sexual identity, appears, as Foucault elaborates in his *History of Sexuality.*[1] But it is important to note that these significant shifts in biomedical discourse and practice around disease and the frequent invocation and citation of biomedical science in juridical practice enabled the biomedical articulation of homosexuality as such. Further, as Dagmar Herzog articulates in *Sexuality in Europe: A Twentieth-Century History*, sexuality was burdened with enormous significance over the course of the twentieth century and acquired growing political salience, given the separation of sexuality from reproduction, which became apparent not only through the rising availability of birth control but also through heightened expectations of pleasure, particularly for women, and a general preoccupation with sexual orientation, sexual rights, and sexual norms (2011, 2-3). In this article, I am interested in interrogating the relationship between scientific opinion as informed by/informing social norms alongside the history of sexual health at particular junctures in the twentieth and twenty-first centuries and the broader politics of gender and sexuality that surround biomedical knowledge.

Given that queer theory functions both as a mode of analysis and as a strategy of opposition that critiques normativities imbricated within a wide range of social categories and social institutions, including, but not limited to the body, gender, healthcare, reproductive politics, the family, and citizenship, in addition to, and alongside, sexuality, my work is shaped by a Foucauldian analysis in situating biomedical discourses on sexuality historically, socially, and culturally in order to analyze their rhetorical appeals to scientific truth and rigor. My analysis here attempts to expose the ways in which gender and sexual health, in biomedical research and practice, is shaped by and shapes prevailing social norms enabled by the historical shifts I have mentioned earlier. Using queer theory as an analytic lens, I would like to explore the implications, contradictions, and collusions at work in discourses surrounding the diagnostic histories and clinical practices around homosexuality that followed the post-war years, the later diagnostic category "Gender Identity Disorder in Childhood" or GIDC, which replaced homosexuality following its removal from the *DSM-III* in 1980, the more recent diagnostic category "Gender Dysphoria in Children" in the current *DSM-V* (American Psychiatric Association 2013), the identification of risk groups for sexually transmitted infections (STIs) such as HIV/AIDS, and the broader politics of gender and sexuality that surround biomedical knowledge.

Nowhere in the clinical literature is the politics of diagnosis more evident than in the history of the listing of homosexuality in the *Diagnostic and Statistical Manual of Mental Disorders* (*DSM*) by the American Psychiatric Association (APA) in the period following the publication of the Kinsey report in 1948 through the historic 1973 decision to delete homosexuality as a diagnostic category. The first edition of the *DSM*, published in 1952, listed homosexuality as psychopathological and as a sociopathic personality disturbance during a time of intense social conformity in the Cold War era. Since the Kinsey report shattered the myth of the effeminate male homosexual and indicated that men with homosexual histories could be found in every age group, social level, occupation, and geographical area (1948, 627), this raised the possibility that gay men could escape detection, and, as Robert Corber argues, linked them with Communists who could conspire to overthrow the US government and subvert its national institutions from within. A resistance to the domestication of gender roles, according to Corber, also raised suspicion toward those men who refused to settle down, raise a family, and take on the roles of breadwinners and homeowners (1997, 11-12). With the rise of social activism in the 1960s against the conflation of homosexuality with mental illness, the *DSM-II*, published in 1968, considered homosexuality as indicative of psychopathology but removed it from the category of sociopathic disturbance, listing it instead under such other "sexual deviations," as fetishism, pedophilia, transvestism, and exhibitionism.[2] Clinical work from this period, especially the ten-year study of the etiology of male homosexuality by Irving Bieber, deliberately shifted psychoanalytic attention away from the role of constitutional factors in the development of homosexuality, which Freud quite adamantly indicated as important to consider,[3] to oedipal and pre-oedipal experiences. The clinical research of this era also promulgated the all-too-familiar stereotype that a high proportion of gay men had "close-binding" mothers who sexually stimulated their sons through over-close intimacy and seductiveness, showed undue concern for their sons' health and safety, and interfered with the relationship of their sons to their fathers and peers, both of whom enable the process of masculine identification through maternal separation (Bieber et al. 1988, 79-81). At the same time, Bieber's study found patterns of prehomosexual childhood as a distinguishing factor of the one hundred six homosexual men studied, compared with the childhoods of one hundred heterosexual men in the control group. Seventy-five percent of men in the homosexual group reported excessive fear of injury in their childhoods, girls as primary playmates in a third of the group, and participation in the "usual" games of boys in less than one-fifth (204). As adults, the homosexual men studied exhibited such behaviors as exaggerated shrugging, "wrist-breaking," lisping, hand-to-hip posturing, and effusiveness, and Bieber reports that these patterns of feminine behavior in males is less an emulation of femininity than a caricature of it, since such behavior in females would appear "bizarre" rather than feminine (188-89). This predates (but ironically addresses) Judith Butler's much later theory of gender as performative and constituted by "the political and cultural intersections in which it is invariably produced and maintained" (1999, 6) through the citation and embodiment of gender norms.

Following intense activism within the medical profession and outside, the American Psychiatric Association set up a committee to review the diagnostic status of homosexuality in the early 1970s, and on the basis of the committee's recommendation, the APA decided to delete homosexuality from the *DSM* in 1973. Rather than signifying the last reference to homosexuality in the official nomenclature of biomedicine, the *DSM-III*, published in 1980, did not contain an entry for homosexuality (except for ego-dystonic homosexuality which was deleted in 1987 in *DSM-III-R*) but added a new diagnostic category "Gender Identity Disorder in Childhood" or GIDC. GIDC, which claimed to align biological sex with the notion of a core gender identity or CGI (see Stoller 1964), has been enforced therapeutically on gender-atypical children, especially boys, who are least capable of resisting it, and treatment for GIDC was often based on the fear of eventual gay outcome. Moreover, the so-called symptoms of GIDC were not remarkably different from those described in earlier research on the etiology of homosexuality in the 1950s and 1960s which served as the intertext for symptomatic descriptions of GIDC in the *DSM-III* (1980) and the *DSM-IV* (APA 1994). Demonstrative of this questionable professed shift from homosexuality to GIDC, Richard Friedman, who chaired the APA Committee which recommended the removal of homosexuality as a diagnostic category from the *DSM*, supported GIDC in his book *Male Homosexuality: A Contemporary Psychoanalytic Perspective* wherein he spoke of gender-atypical boys as having "female-like symptoms" (1988, 199) and argued that most childhood effeminacy results in homosexuality and that most adult homosexuality is preceded by some kind of prepubertal *gender disturbance* (212).

Additionally, as with the earlier research on homosexuality, Susan Coates and Kenneth Zucker, internationally-known experts on GIDC, have described mothers of feminine boys as overbearing and pathogenic through transferring their unresolved trauma on to their sons. For Coates and Person, for example, this suggests a "disturbed" mother-child interaction and that boyhood femininity is symptomatic of separation anxiety and a desire "to restore a fantasy tie to the physically or emotionally absent mother" (708). As with the earlier work on homosexuality, mothers are blamed for the gender nonconformity of their sons. In the years leading up to the publications of the *DSM-V*, LGBTQ activists opposed vehemently Kenneth Zucker's appointment by the APA in 2008 to chair the workgroup on Gender and Sexual Identity Disorders for the next edition of the *DSM* largely because of his work on gender identity disorder in children. In 2015, Zucker's Gender Identity Disorder Clinic, part of the Toronto Centre for Addiction and Mental Health (CAMH), was closed. Following an external review critical of the way the clinic treated children and young patients struggling with issues related to their gender identity, Zucker's dismissal, according to the Toronto *Globe and Mail*, was a result of his work no longer being "in step with the latest thinking" given that it suggested that gender nonconforming children be discouraged from becoming transgender adults, which many in the transgender community viewed as a form of conversion therapy (Anderseen 2016).

The current *DSM-V* replaces the diagnostic category GIDC with "Gender Dysphoria" with a separate section dedicated to children, signifying the further displacement of the diagnostic category rather than its disappearance. It describes gender dysphoria as a marked incongruence between one's experienced/expressed gender and one's assigned gender, the latter of which is based on, and conflated with, natal sex. The diagnostic criteria include a child's strong preference for the clothing of the other gender; a strong preference for cross-gender roles in make-believe or fantasy play and for the toys, games, and pastimes more typical for the other gender; and the attendant stress that accompanies such incongruence (APA 2013). While the *DSM* now stipulates that the term "gender dysphoria" is more descriptive than the previous usage of "gender identity disorder" as it related to children in the previous editions (APA 2013), the diagnostic criteria for gender dysphoria in children, and the attendant descriptors, seem remarkably similar to those for GIDC, and still echo, to some degree, earlier work on the etiology of homosexuality with regard to its tropes in describing gender variance in children.[4]

What the diagnostic history of homosexuality, GIDC, and gender dysphoria in children point to is to the ways in which biomedical knowledge is structured around the polarity of the normal and the pathological to the extent that all have served to maintain heteronormative gender norms. This discursive formation supports Judith Butler's claim that sexuality in culture "is regulated through the policing and the shaming of gender" (1993, 238) while providing a powerful and legitimate discursive and clinical apparatus for that very shaming and policing and its medical and social reinforcement. Moreover, these instantiations of homophobia, transphobia, and misogyny in the clinical literature, past and ongoing, have not only been condoned biomedically and clinically but continue to provoke social condemnation, discrimination, the incitement to violence, and the bullying of children who cross-gender identify, with higher rates of suicide among them, in addition to various form of social exclusion, actual or imagined, against gender nonconforming children and gender and sexual dissidents more broadly, while continuing to undermine erotic autonomy and gender expression as fundamental human rights. In addition, mothers have been pathologized in clinical literature as overprotective, indulgent, seductive, overanxious, or unhappily married, and not the slightest consideration has been given to the possibility for mother's and son's subjectivities affording greater closeness and empathy (Corbett 1999, 129). Moreover, to what extent will a clinical diagnosis of gender dysphoria in a child be related to a fear of possible gay outcome by therapists, medical professionals, and parents? As I have written previously, what also needs to be pointed out is that transgender identification in children points to the failure of the matrix of heterosexuality to legislate itself fully. In these post-theoretical, post-queer times, how can the trans rupture in the matrix of gender intelligibility be welcomed as producing new identificatory sites and new conceptual apparatuses for understanding the psychological growth of children who cross-gender identify (who may or may not turn out to be gay) and LGBTQ people (who may or may not conform to prescribed gender norms) (Spurlin 1998, 91)?

Another site that encapsulates the regulation of biomedicine through the vicissitudes of social normativities lies in the history of the HIV/AIDS pandemic. Early manifestations of AIDS-related illnesses exposed a gap in biomedical knowledge and thinking in the early 1980s when gay men were identified as a primary risk group and as primary carriers of the virus, without a clear understanding of the epidemiological foundations of HIV/AIDS. Before the isolation of the human immunodeficiency virus, and certainly after, biomedical science contributed to the emergence of new discourses of sexual perversion centered on metaphors of social defiance, erotic indulgence, hedonism, and moral laxity around the transmission of HIV either sexually or through shared needles used intravenously. Ironically, this was right at the same time that the *DSM-III* (the first edition of the *DSM* not to list homosexuality as mental disorder) was published, so that homosexuality became once again, but differentially, cast as a perversion. Those who were diagnosed with HIV seropositivity, as Susan Sontag notes, were cast as deserving of blame (1989, 26) to the extent that gay men, intravenous drug users, and those of Haitian descent were seen as "disposable" groups and the primary risk groups for acquiring HIV in the United States. As Cindy Patton observes, the pandemic gained its social meaning over time by building on already deeply seated social prejudices surrounding race, class, gender, sexuality, and addiction. Those who suffered the specter of decadence, decay, and death associated with HIV/AIDS, she argues, were seen initially as isolated cases, which helped to erase the social realities that shaped the growing epidemic (1990, 25). "Good health" in the early days of HIV/AIDS was defined by the medical profession, social health policy, and the media through such vectors as whiteness, western location, rationality, emotional self-control, and middle-class values such as hard work, productivity, and moderate habits as safeguards against licentiousness, sexual indulgence, and addictive behaviors that would lead to decadence and disease, not remarkably different from the codes of bourgeois morality that shaped rising nationalisms in late eighteenth-century Europe. This points not only to racial and class hierarchies in understanding HIV/AIDS in the early 1980s but also substantiates the fact that biomedical knowledge is always already mediated and produced through and around particular cultural symbols (Patton 1990, 67) and that the scientific authority it holds has been used politically as a form of sanctioned governance to incite and perpetuate discriminatory social practices.

In considering an important historical precedent, biomedical discourses on sexuality were closely linked to the racial politics of National Socialism, whereby Nazi doctors studied homosexuality as a form of social degeneracy and as a threat to racial hygiene, appealing to the authority of biomedical science in order to maintain rigid social distinctions between the genders and the procreative responsibility of Aryan citizens. In the mid-1930s, medical doctors in Germany argued nearly unanimously that homosexuality, medically speaking, was a threat to public health; Germany's leading public health journal at the time *Der Öffentliche Gesundheitsdienst* described homosexuality as a psychopathology (Proctor 1988, 212),[5] not that far removed from clinical descriptions of homosexuality in the *DSM-I* nearly twenty years later. Arguing against homosexuality as biologically determined, one Nazi doctor, in writing for the Reich Office of Racial Policy in 1938, proclaimed that homosexuals, like Jews, were state criminals and "not 'poor, sick' people to be treated, but enemies of the state to be eliminated" (Proctor 1988, 213).[6] Going back further, Mosse and others have noted that late nineteenth-century medical literature in Europe, very much influenced by scientific racism at the time, often conflated the pathologies of male Jews and homosexuals—both were thought to be prone to hysteria, nervous bodily distortions, and feminine tone of voice and bodily movements (1999, 64).[7]

The biomedicalization of homosexuality under National Socialism was by no means a momentary aberration as nationalist discourses in much of the postcolonial world today read homosexuality as a colonial import and as a form of western decadence that is foreign to indigenous cultural traditions. Western biomedicine has played a role historically as a tool of imperial power. Frantz Fanon, an early postcolonial theorist originally from Martinique who studied medicine and psychiatry in France, and served a medical residency in Algeria and became involved in Algeria's struggle for independence, noted that medical knowledge was one of the most insidious tools of colonial conquest and contributed to the dehumanizing logic of colonial rule (1963, 296). Similarly speaking of the French colonial conquest of Algeria, Richard Keller notes in *Colonial Madness* that physicians, surgeons, and pharmacists saw diagnosis and treatment as a contest over civilization alongside health and disease (2007, 11). In terms of sexuality, this meant that European physicians in the late nineteenth and early twentieth centuries read Africa in particular as "a space of savage violence and lurid sexuality" (1). Largely as a result of the effects of the so-called civilizing mission of colonialism, and the remnants of homophobic laws that often have their origins in colonial administration, HIV/AIDS sufferers in many postcolonial societies today bear the stigma of sexual deviance and moral laxity, and these markings have been shaped by a history of imperialism, outdated western psychiatric opinion on the etiology of homosexuality, and causal links between homosexuality and HIV/AIDS constructed by western biomedicine in the early history of the pandemic. Yet the effects of the biomedical justification of colonial rule continue in the contemporary surveillance and tracking of HIV/AIDS by global health institutions such as the World Health Organization (WHO) and UNAIDS. As Cindy Patton has argued, the term "African AIDS," used early in the pandemic, mobilized racist ideologies of unchecked, unbridled sexuality amongst indigenous Africans and amongst blacks in general.[8] The rhetorical strategies of medical thought-styles in representations of HIV/AIDS globally, Patton notes, have been deeply layered with social ideologies around race, class, and sexuality, and have the power "to structure the terms through which bodies become visible as the locations of disease, of an epidemic" (2002, 26).

Another problem with the effects of imperialism was the initial reluctance of many African nations to admit to a presence of homosexuality within their borders and even higher rates of HIV infection than were originally assumed or predicted. This was tied to deep-seated historical anxieties about discursive appropriations of African sexuality by the West in decadent terms, a legacy of colonialism which remains, as with the term "African AIDS," in discourses surrounding the global surveillance and tracking of HIV/AIDS. At the same time, the reading of homosexuality as un-African by some strands of African cultural nationalism produced a significant gap for those at risk for HIV who escaped the categories of the West, given that some indigenous African men practiced anal sex with other men but did not identify as gay and lived heterosexual lives publicly, which was compounded by the fact that the WHO saw HIV transmission in Africa largely in heterosexual terms in the early days of the pandemic. AIDS educators were not initially sensitive to the fact that anal sex has different meanings and values in different cultural systems that needed to be addressed in helping those men, who engaged in the practice of anal sex with other men as partners, recognize that safer sex applied to them as well, even if they resisted taking on a gay identity as it is understood in the West. The adoption of the descriptive phrase "men who have sex with men," or MSM, by the WHO's Global Programme on AIDS provided a thinly veiled screen, or closet, at the time, not of mere secrecy but of a "safe" identity that was more legibly heterosexual but later, it was realized, no less at risk for HIV transmission or infection. The problem with western understandings of homosexuality, initially imposed by global health organizations on indigenous men who have sex with men, was not so much the conflation of anal sex with homosexuality but the conflation of sexual *practice* with sexual *identity*, which places Foucault's proposition of a shift in homosexuality in the nineteenth century from a temporary aberration to an emergent identic category (1980, 42-43) even more firmly in the West. More important, such imperialist thinking missed significant forms of HIV transmission not immediately apparent to western thinking, which was based on the confluence of sexual practice with sexual identity and resulted in subsequent gaps and delays in education and prevention programs in large parts of sub-Sahara Africa early in the pandemic.

Additionally, placid assumptions in the West that the availability of anti-retroviral (ARV) medication no longer signifies eventual death for those who are HIV-positive fail to recognize that this is precisely what it does signify for the many indigenous Africans in sub-Sahara Africa dying from AIDS-related illnesses each day. South Africa has the highest prevalence of HIV/AIDS in the world, estimated by the South African government's statistical report of 2015 to be at about 6.19 million of its total population of 54.96 million with the highest impact of HIV/AIDS falling on indigenous African women (Statistics South Africa 2015). A report on violence against women and HIV/AIDS by the UNAIDS Coalition on Women and AIDS and the WHO points to the everyday realities of gender inequality and intimate partner violence in South Africa. It is difficult for women, particularly younger women, to negotiate condom use with intimate male partners. High rates of gender-based violence and rape often serve as barriers to women seeking HIV testing, anti-retroviral treatment, and access to services which could prevent mother to child transmission (UNAIDS Global Coalition on Women and AIDS and WHO 2005). Alarming numbers of indigenous African women who identify as lesbian experience "corrective rape" as a cure for their so-called aberrant desires, placing them at risk for HIV/AIDS as well.

Another issue pointing to the high prevalence of HIV/AIDS in South Africa is that in the late 1990s and in the early part of the last decade, some global health officials argued that those living in poverty were not literate enough to follow the prescribed regimen of treatment for taking ARV medication; this racist argument, in turn, was appropriated by western pharmaceutical companies as a rationale for not lowering the cost of the drugs so that they would be affordable to poorer South Africans, arguing that a failure to take the drugs responsibly could lead to drug-resistant strains of HIV. The Treatment Action Campaign (TAC) in South Africa has been the most vocal and visible lobby fighting for the rights of HIV-positive people for equal access to treatment; in the late 1990s, TAC willfully ignored international trade agreements pertaining to the production, import, and use of less costly generic versions of patented ARV drugs for the treatment of HIV infection. More recently, TAC has put pressure on UNAIDS not to overstate the likelihood of ending HIV/AIDS given the deleterious effects this could have on donorship for global HIV/AIDS funding and the politics of sexual healthcare in the developing world. The French nongovernmental human rights organization, Médecins Sans Frontières/Doctors without Borders, has worked in some of the most impoverished townships in South Africa providing ARV and TB medication to those living with HIVAIDS who are facing the challenges of poverty, marginalization, and stigma. Their work defies earlier biomedical discourses on HIV/AIDS in Africa purporting that poor Africans were too uneducated to take the medications responsibly. Given South Africa's history of disobedience, struggle, and resistance to oppressive regimes, this work calls attention to the production and distribution of power which certainly is imbricated with biomedical thinking around ARV access and pricing in the developing world.

In conclusion, if sexual desire can become a mechanism for various forms of social manipulation, how does western biomedicine continue to play a significant political role in the cultural management of gender and sexual norms? How might the relationship between the clinical and cultural spheres be better engaged in biomedical knowledge and practice, especially around the topic of sexual health, given biomedicine's historic failure to recognize the influence of homophobia and transphobia in, and their reproduction through, the diagnostic histories of homosexuality and GIDC, and the racial, gender, class, and sexual ideologies that constructed early readings of the HIV/AIDS pandemic in the West and in the postcolonial world? While the identification of risk groups is key for understanding patterns of disease transmission, especially in the case of HIV/AIDS in the context of sexual health, and is essential to helping people to avoid becoming ill, what social and cultural ideologies are operating in epidemiological discourses about specific risk groups and their behavior? Where will this theorization occur?

What the diagnostic histories and medicalizations of homosexuality, gender identity disorder, gender dysphoria, and HIV/AIDS also indicate is a link between compulsory heterosexuality and compulsory able-bodiedness as theorized in contemporary disability studies. As Robert McRuer argues, medically speaking, the ideal heterosexual subject is one whose sexuality is not compromised by disability such as queerness; whereas the ideal or successful able-bodied subject is one whose ability is not compromised by queerness, that is, by disability (2010, 387). As evident from the earlier discussion, medical science historically has seen the queer body as a disabled or diseased body, and the remnants of colonial medicine that operated in the early days of the HIV/AIDS pandemic held the white, western, heterosexual body as the standard of normality and health. These links are important since biomedicine as a discipline, and as a form of knowledge production, addresses various forms of disability and disease but historically without a theorization of the cultural politics that dictate, in this context, the ways in which "compulsory heterosexuality is contingent on compulsory able-bodiedness and vice versa" (McRuer 2010, 384), and, more broadly, the social and cultural conditions that inform the normal/pathological split.[9]

The ongoing heteronormative slant in medical education in North America and elsewhere is certainly not promising; studies have shown that specific healthcare issues pertaining to lesbian, gay, bisexual, and transgendered patients are not being adequately addressed in clinical training, pointing to a cultural blind spot, another instantiation of the normal/

pathological binary, and a refusal to engage with the exceptions and contingencies of what is prescribed as normative. What are the social repercussions for critical healing? A study by the Stanford University School of Medicine, published in September 2011 in *JAMA*, found that students at one-third of 176 responding medical schools in the United States and Canada received *no* gay-related healthcare education during their clinical years; only three in five schools provided instruction in eight or more of the sixteen health issues of concern to lesbian, gay, bisexual, or transgendered people, including sex reassignment surgery, inaccessibility to healthcare, safer sex, and chronic (sexual) disease.[10] A more recent study on implicit bias against sexual minorities in biomedicine, published in *Academic Medicine* in 2015, found that 46% of heterosexual first-year medical students in the US expressed some explicit bias against lesbians and gay men and that 82% held implicit biases; that is, they held ingrained, but unrecognized or unconscious, beliefs toward the target group (Fallin-Bennett 2015, 549). The study recognizes that further work needs to show that biases such as these actually affect LGBT patient care, but other studies have shown that implicit racial bias, for example, does affect physician decision making, and that it is reasonable to assume that LGBT patients are also at risk for discrimination and compromised care in the biomedical context (549). A study published in *Virtual Mentor* the previous year by Jonathan Metzl and Dorothy E. Roberts found that extra-clinical stigma, socioeconomic factors, and cultural politics shape diagnostic and treatment disparities just as these similarly shape the material realities of patients' lives. African-Americans were much more likely to receive diagnoses for schizophrenia as compared with white patients but less likely to be diagnosed with depression or bipolar disorders compared with their white counterparts (Metzl and Roberts 2014, 675). The article asks that the clinical situation be understood as constructed by political, economic, racial, and gendered social structures and hierarchies that produce vulnerability for particular groups of patients (682).

Yet, while it appears as if their analysis is demonstrating the ways in which cultural politics construct the clinical situation and the dynamics of patient care, Metzl and his colleagues fail to account for clinical attitudes toward sexuality as a significant vector of influence. In theorizing medical engagement with stigma and inequality in an article on structural competency in medical education, published in *Social Sciences and Medicine*, also in 2014, Metzl and Hansen argue that medical education needs to train health care professionals more systematically so that they can think about how such variables as race, social class, gender, and ethnicity shape and are shaped by the interactions between doctors and patients (Metzl and Hansen 2014, 127). It is no wonder that the development of structural competency in medical education seems to occlude sexuality, as it does so again here, given that 40% of physicians in the US reported in 2010 as to having no training in LGBT health in medical school or in their residencies (Fallin-Bennett 2015, 550). In addition, remnant homophobia in medical workplaces and schools, especially evident through homophobic remarks, has resulted in a reluctance for medical providers to come out. Fallin-Bennett cites a 2011 study by Mansh and White on the experiences of LGBT medical students, which was presented at the American Association of Medical Colleges annual conference; in the study, 16-17% of lesbians and gay men, 50% of bisexuals, and 60% of those who were transgendered did not disclose their sexual or gender identities in contexts related to medical school in the US (Mansh and White 2011; in Fallin-Bennett 2015, 550). In addition, Fallin-Bennett surmises, while acknowledging that this requires further study, that LGBT students may be more likely than their heterosexual or gender-conforming peers not to apply to medical school or to drop out once they are there (2015, 550).

With implicit and explicit bias toward them in medical and clinical settings, LGBT patients feel reluctant to come out to their medical providers for fear of discrimination and judgment given that these biases seem to be ignored, if not reinforced, in medical education and clinical training, which can negatively affect the quality of care received by LGBT patients. Historically, this may be because biomedicine has produced highly advanced knowledge of the biological impacts of lived environments with relatively undertheorized analyses of the environments themselves and their social and cultural impacts on medical decisions and patient care (Metzl and Hansen 2014, 129). Yet it is also historical to point out, as I have been arguing in this article, that healthcare systems and individual practitioners and researchers have systematically pathologized homosexuality and gender nonconformity, the latter most recently in children. As a result, LGBTQI patients have often undergone reparative conversion therapies, which have now been deemed inappropriate and harmful, and children born with DSD, or disorders in sex development, have been subjected to invasive and damaging interventions, including hormonal treatments and genital cosmetic surgery. More generally, and even without specific "corrective" treatments, the lingering, and still all-too-present actual, internalized, and anticipated medical and social stigmas experienced by LGBTQI people often result in risky behaviors amongst those in this vulnerable group that create significant disparities in their physical and mental health (Eckstrand and Sciolla 2014, 12, 14). It is important to note that the annual report of the United Nations Human Rights Council, published by the United Nations High Commissioner for Human Rights and entitled "Discrimination and violence against individuals based on their sexual orientation and gender identity," stipulates quite clearly that conversion therapy and gender reassignment, when forced or involuntary, as well as unnecessary medical interventions involving intersex children, break the UN's prohibition on torture (UN High Commissioner for Human Rights 2015, 11). Moreover, as I have been arguing, the Report also stipulates that discriminatory policies and practices of healthcare institutions adversely affect the quality of health services and deter patients from seeking them (UN High Commissioner for Human Rights 2015, 14). This implies radical analyses of new kinds of interventions, contestations, and struggles around the conflation of good health with conformity to gender and sexual norms, as well as further analysis into the contradictions between the urgency of ethical biomedical practice and critical healing alongside the various discourses, ideologies, and cultures which shape biomedicine, and by which biomedical knowledge and clinical practices are themselves shaped.

Endnotes

[1] See Foucault 1980, 42-43 *History of Sexuality.*

[2] For psychoanalytic work on homosexuality from this early period, from the late 1940s through 1970, see Sandor Rado, 1949; Edmund Bergler, 1956; Bieber, et al., 1962, *Homosexuality: A Psychoanalytic Study of Male Homosexuals,* New York: Basic Books, reprinted as Irving Bieber, et al., 1988, *Homosexuality: A Psychoanalytic Study,* Northvale, NJ: Aronson; and Charles Socarides, 1968.

[3] In his *Three Essays on the Theory of Sexuality,* Freud remarks that "the exclusive sexual interest felt by men for women is also a problem that needs elucidating and is not a self-evident fact based upon an attraction that is ultimately of a chemical nature. A person's final sexual attitude is not decided until after puberty and is the result of a number of factors, not all of which are yet known; some are of a constitutional nature but others are accidental" (Freud 1962, n1, 12).

[4] While the connection to the medicalization of gender has already been discussed in Bieber's work on the etiology of homosexuality in the post-war years, the descriptions of GIDC in the *DSM-III* and *DSM-IV* list such diagnostic criteria as a preference for cross-dressing or simulating female attire in boys, an insistence on wearing only stereotypically masculine clothing in girls; strong and persistent preferences for cross-sex roles in make-believe play or persistent fantasies of being the other sex; intense desires to participate in the stereotypical games and pastimes of the other sex, and a strong preference for playmates of the other sex (APA 1994, 537). The *DSM-V* does stipulate that the clinical problem is on dysphoria and not on gender identity per se (APA 2013).

[5] For the German language text to which Proctor is referring, see J. Lange, 1938.

[6] For the German source to which Proctor refers, see "Staatsfeinde sind auszumerzen!" *Informationsdienst*, June 20, 1938.

[7] As I have argued elsewhere, the social use of biomedical discourses relegated homosexuals under National Socialism as threats to the economic and political well-being of the German nation-state, and played a role in justifying persecutions against them, including the revision of Paragraph 175 of the Reich Penal Code. See Spurlin, 2009, *Lost Intimacies: Rethinking Homosexuality under National Socialism*, especially Chapters 2 and 3.

[8] For example, an article on HIV/AIDS in southern Africa in *The Economist* in 2002 begins with a voyeuristic narrative of sexual practices in Botswana, describing some indigenous men's preferences for "dry sex" whereby women, in order to provide more pleasure for their male partners, insert toothpaste or herbs into their vaginas in order to prevent lubrication, which can lead to tears in vaginal tissues and bleeding during penetration and thereby allow the human immunodeficiency virus to penetrate the tissue. While the practice, provided the male partner is HIV-infected, can place the woman at risk for infection, beginning an article about HIV/AIDS in southern Africa with "dry sex" reproduces textually an orientalist erotics that imagines non-western exotic otherness as a site of sexual deviance or excess, supposedly far removed from the sexual epistemologies and practices of the West. See "Fighting Back. Special Report: AIDS in Southern Africa" 2002.

[9] McRuer also links able-bodied identity and heterosexual identity as performative given that each identity "is simultaneously the ground on which all identities supposedly rest (as natural, as given) and an impressive achievement that is always deferred and thus never really guaranteed" (2010, 386; parentheses mine). This calls to mind Butler's theory of gender performativity through the citation and embodiment of gender norms, which creates the illusion of gender as a substance of being instead of as "a complexity whose totality is permanently deferred, never fully what it is at any given juncture in time' (Butler 1999, 22).

[10] As examples, the study indicated that cervical cancer and genital human papillomavirus often go untreated in lesbians, high rates of hepatitis remain high among gay men, and transgendered individuals who take unprescribed hormones in the later stages of gender transitioning risk infection and other side effects. See Juno Obedin-Maliver, Elizabeth S. Goldsmith, Leslie Stewart, et al., 2011.

References

American Psychiatric Association (APA). 1994. *The Diagnostic and Statistical Manual of Mental Disorders*. 4th edition. Washington, DC: American Psychiatric Association.

——. 2013. *The Diagnostic and Statistical Manual of Mental Disorders*. 5th edition. Washington DC: American Psychiatric Association. https://doi.org/10.1176/appi.books.9780890425596.dms14.

Anderscen, Erin. 2016. "Gender Identity Debate Swirls over CAMH Psychologist, Transgender Program." *The Globe and Mail*. February 14. http://www.theglobeandmail.com/news/toronto/gender-identity-debate-swirls-over-camh-psychologist-transgender-program/article28758828/.

Bergler, Edmund. 1956, *Homosexuality: Disease or Way of Life?*, New York: Hill and Wang;

Bieber, Irving, et al. (1962) 1988. *Homosexuality: A Psychoanalytic Study*. Northvale, NJ: Aronson.

 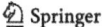

Butler, Judith. (1990) 1999. *Gender Trouble: Feminism and the Subversion of Identity*. New York: Routledge.

———. 1993. *Bodies that Matter: On the Discursive Limits of 'Sex'*. New York: Routledge.

Coates, Susan and Ethel Spector Person. 1985. "Extreme boyhood femininity: Isolated behavior or pervasive disorder?" *Journal of the American Academy of Child and Adolescent Psychiatry* 24.6: 702-709.

Corber, Robert J. 1997. *Homosexuality in Cold War America: Resistance and the Crisis of Masculinity*. Durham: Duke University Press.

Corbett, Ken. 1999. "Homosexual Boyhood: Notes on Girlyboys." In *Sissies and Tomboys: Gender Nonconformity and Homosexual Childhood*, edited by Matthew Rottek, 107-139. New York: New York University Press.

Eckstrand, Kristen L. and Andrés F. Sciolla. 2014. "History of Health Disparities Among Individuals Who Are or May Be LGBT, Gender Nonconforming, and/or Born with DSD." In *Implementing Curricular and Institutional Climate Changes to Improve Health Care for Individuals Who Are LGBT, Gender Nonconforming, or Born with DSD*, 10-21. Washington, DC: Association of American Medical Colleges.

Fallin-Bennett, Keisa. 2015. "Implicit Bias against Sexual Minorities in Medicine: Cycle of Professional Influence and the Role of the Hidden Curriculum." *Academic Medicine* 90 (5): 549-552.

Fanon, Frantz. 1963. *The Wretched of the Earth*. Translated by Constance Farrington. New York: Grove Press.

"Fighting Back. 2002. Special Report: AIDS in Southern Africa." *The Economist*. May 11: 27-29.

Foucault, Michel. (1963) 1973. *The Birth of the Clinic: An Archaeology of Medical Perception*. Translated by A.M. Sheridan Smith. New York: Vintage.

———. (1976) 1980. *The History of Sexuality, Volume I: An Introduction*. Translated by Robert Hurley. New York: Vintage.

Freud, Sigmund. 1962. *Three Essays on the Theory of Sexuality*. Translated by James Strachey. New York: Basic Books.

Friedman, Richard C. 1988. *Male Homosexuality: A Contemporary Psychoanalytic Perspective*. New Haven: Yale University Press.

Herzog, Dagmar. 2011. *Sexuality in Europe: A Twentieth-Century History*. Cambridge: Cambridge University Press.

Keller, Richard C. 2007. *Colonial Madness: Psychiatry in French North Africa*. Chicago: University of Chicago Press.

Kinsey, Alfred C., et al. 1948. *Sexual Behavior in the Human Male*. Philadelphia: W.B. Saunders.

Lange, J. 1938. "Die Feststellung und Wertung geistiger Störungen im Ehegesundheitsgesetz," *Öffentlicher Gesundheitsdienst* 4: 533.

Mansh, M. and W. White. 2011. "Lesbian, Gay, Bisexual, and Transgender Medical Student Experiences: 'Out' in Medical School and Perspectives on Curricular Content." Poster Presentation. Annual Meeting of the Association of American Medical Colleges. Denver.

McRuer, Robert. 2010. "Compulsory Able-Bodiedness and Queer/Disabled Existence." In *The Disability Studies Reader*, edited by Lennard J. Davis, 3rd edition, 383-392. New York: Routledge.

Metzl, Jonathan M. and Helena Hansen. 2014. "Structural Competency: Theorizing a New Medical Engagement with Stigma and Inequality." *Social Science & Medicine* 103: 126-133.

Metzl, Jonathan M. and Dorothy E. Roberts. 2014. "Structural Competency Meets Structural Racism: Race, Politics, and the Structure of Medical Knowledge." *Virtual Mentor: American Medical Association Journal of Ethics* 16 (9): 674-690.

Mosse George. 1999. *The Fascist Revolution: Toward a General Theory of Fascism*. New York: Howard Fertig.

Obedin-Maliver, June, Elizabeth S. Goldsmith, Leslie Stewart, et al. 2011. "Lesbian, Gay, Bisexual, and Transgender-Related Content in Undergraduate Medical Education." *JAMA* 306 (9): 971-977.

Parker, Andrew, Mary Russo, et al, eds. 1992. *Nationalisms and Sexualities*. New York: Routledge.

Patton, Cindy. 1990. *Inventing AIDS*. New York: Routledge.

———. 2002. *Globalizing AIDS*. Minneapolis: University of Minnesota Press.

Proctor, Robert N. 1988. *Racial Hygiene: Medicine under the Nazis*. Cambridge, MA: Harvard University Press.

Rado, Sandor. 1949, "An Adaptational View of Sexual Behavior." *Psychosexual Development in Health and Disease*, Eds. P. Hoch and J. Zubin, 159-189. New York: Grune and Stratton.

Socarides, Charles. 1968, *The Overt Homosexual*, New York: Grune and Stratton.

Sontag, Susan. 1989. *AIDS and Its Metaphors*. New York: Farrar, Straus and Giroux.

Spurlin, William J. 1998. "Sissies and Sisters: Gender, Sexuality and the Possibilities of Coalition." In *Coming Out of Feminism?*, edited by Mandy Merck, Naomi Segal, and Elizabeth Wright, 74-101. Oxford: Blackwell.

———. 2009. *Lost Intimacies: Rethinking Homosexuality under National Socialism*. New York: Lang Publishing.

Statistics South Africa Report, 2015. South African Government. https://www.statssa.gov.za/publications/P0302/P03022015.pdf.

Stoller, Robert J. 1964. "A Contribution to the Study of Gender Identity." *International Journal of Psychoanalysis* 45: 220-226.

UNAIDS Global Coalition on Women and AIDS and WHO. 2005. "Violence against Women and HIV/AIDS: Critical Intersections. Intimate Partner Violence and HIV/AIDS." World Health Organization. http://www.who.int/hac/techguidance/pht/InfoBulletinIntimatePartnerViolenceFinal.pdf.

United Nations High Commissioner for Human Rights. 2015. "Discrimination and Violence against Individuals Based on their Sexual Orientation and Gender Identity." New York: General Assembly and Human Rights Council of the United Nations. 4 May.

J Med Humanit (2019) 40:21–31
https://doi.org/10.1007/s10912-018-9524-2

Choir Boy: Trans Vocal Performance and the De-Pathologization of Transition

Marty Fink[1]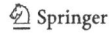

Published online: 11 July 2018
© Springer Science+Business Media, LLC, part of Springer Nature 2018

Abstract This paper will examine *Choir Boy* (2005), a trans coming-of-age novel by Charlie Anders, to disrupt historically rooted medical narratives of gender transition. Through a disability studies lens, this paper locates vocal performance as a means of speaking back to gatekeeping practices held in place by medical authorities since the inception of transsexuality as a classificatory category. Offering imaginative alternatives to "wrong body" diagnostics, this analysis places cultural texts in conversation with disability theory to reframe the trans self as a singing body that cannot be reduced to normalizing biomedical practices. *Choir Boy* frames vocal performance as a mode of gender expression and as a survival strategy against violence. The trans counter-narratives offered by Anders resist the medicalization of trans bodies and the classification of some bodies as not "trans enough" to qualify for transition. *Choir Boy* locates vocal performance and not binary gender identification as impetus for transition, thereby advocating for trans self-determination over medical access.

Keywords Trans · Queer · Gender · Transition · Gatekeeping

A false case: re-scripting wrong body narratives

In 1954, Doctor Harry Benjamin published a set of diagnostic criteria by which individuals could be medically labeled as transsexuals. It was through this clinical diagnosis of transsexuality that individuals could gain corresponding access to gender-confirming healthcare such as surgeries and hormone therapy. Medical access not only altered trans individuals' physical bodies but also granted access to necessary administrative paperwork such as accurate gender markers on identification documents required to attain jobs, housing, and social services (Stryker 2005). Having a gender

✉ Marty Fink
  marty.fink@ryerson.ca

[1] Ryerson University, 350 Victoria Street, Toronto, ON M5B 2K3, Canada

presentation that does not match the gender marker that appears on one's birth certificate or driver's license not merely provided barriers to resource access in the 1950s but also continues to prohibit trans people—especially those facing intersecting oppressions—from accessing employment, educational, and housing opportunities today (Spade 2011). Grassroots organizers and academics have since confronted the reductive nature of such diagnostic practices by exposing the fault lines of their logic: if a community of trans people know which narratives to tell about being in the wrong body in order to access gender-confirming healthcare and the administrative access it unlocks, these medically defined narratives of trans-ness become both culturally prevalent ways of understanding trans experiences as well as culturally necessary tropes to resist. This paper will examine *Choir Boy* (2005), a trans coming-of-age novel by Charlie Anders, to disrupt the ongoing biomedical stronghold on narratives of transition. Offering imaginative alternatives to wrong body diagnostics, this novel reframes the trans self as a singing body that cannot be reduced to normalizing classificatory practices. Through an investigation of trans medical history, disability studies, and vocal performance in *Choir Boy,* this paper will suggest alternatives to biomedical, psychological, and administrative gatekeeping, advocating instead for the self-determination of trans embodiment and medical access.

Choir Boy presents the story of pre-adolescent Berry who wants so wholeheartedly to remain a star in his church choir that he secretly begins taking hormones to allay the vocal interference of puberty. Berry soon finds himself faced with the demand to declare a gender identity that corresponds with his now-modified body and still-treble singing capacities. Following a meeting with the school principal forcing Berry to commit to a gender to live in at school, Berry's mother confronts him with a hard and fast choice between male and female identity: "So what's it going to be, Berry? What are you?" To this, Berry can only reply, "I'm a choirboy" (268). Given the limiting options of male and female, Berry asserts a form of self-definition that is bound not by binary gender identification but by the performative expression of voice.

Anders's narrative rendering of Berry's vocal identification accordingly draws on the contours of voice to speak back to (sing back to) the biomedical gatekeeping of adolescent gender embodiment. In a session with his psychologist, Berry sits silently and refuses to talk, his vocals resisting psychotherapeutic and service provider scripts of pathologization. Rather than simply accepting his role as patient by reciting the prescribed narrative of "wrong body" entrapment, Berry "opened his mouth and music came out. He hadn't decided to sing in therapy, but once it happened it seemed a good thing. Once the trained voice flowed, Berry felt in control of the situation for the first time" (47). Berry's "trained" voice challenges the power dynamic between healthcare professionals and care recipients who are positioned as holding less knowledge about their own bodies and medical needs than the gatekeepers upon whom they depend for access to care. Berry quickly learns from his trans peers that receiving access to hormones requires adopting the wrong body narrative, the storyline that "this shell doesn't represent me, I'm making my way through this world in a false case" (57). Berry is advised that he must express to his doctors sentiments such as "you hate your manhood. Your body blows chunks. You were born the wrong shape" (60). In using the clinical arena to showcase his own expertise through the act of singing, Berry positions his gender identity not within these conventional medicalized narratives expected of him but in relation to the preservation of his voice.

Wronged bodies: the medicalization of trans identity

Berry's experience of learning about the wrong body narrative and how to adopt it in order to receive access to his medical needs reflects a long history of the provider-patient dynamics around which trans identity is understood. Although trans people have always existed, transsexual identities, as cultural scholars have noted, were first defined alongside the modern invention of sexual reassignment surgery in the mid-twentieth century. In the US, it was not until access to hormones and surgical procedures required medical gatekeeping criteria that the category of the "transsexual" gained a set of narrative and diagnostic features (Meyerowitz 2002, 4). Such features served first to pathologize and then to "treat" and "correct" individuals already occupying a variety of gender nonconforming practices. As Sandy Stone outlines in "The Empire Strikes Back: A Posttranssexual Manifesto" (1991, 291), retelling narratives about being a woman trapped in man's body became cultural currency and medical convention, as patients presenting this narrative were granted medical access and the administrative benefits that followed. Stone observes that "the reason candidates' behavioral profiles matched Benjamin's so well was that the candidates, too, had read Benjamin's book, which was passed from hand to hand within the transsexual community, and they were only too happy to provide the behavior that led to acceptance for surgery."

This oft-referenced clinical treatment manual, *The Transsexual Phenomenon* (Benjamin 1966), effectively opened up a medical pathway for trans women in the US to gain the clinical and administrative support they needed to live in their correct gender identities. In *Whipping Girl: A Transsexual Woman on Sexism and the Scapegoating of Femininity,* Julia Serano (2007, 118) exposes Benjamin's book as flawed in its hierarchical rating of some trans women as "true transsexuals" in opposition to those he classified as "pseudo transvestites," categories that affirmed the trans-ness of some trans women and not others. Serano also details the impact of this inaugural medical gatekeeping system through which doctors and not trans people themselves are positioned as authorities on whether or not someone is trans enough to be trans; nevertheless, Serano credits Benjamin for recognizing the large variation that exists among trans women, as the book acknowledges that not everyone who is trans or gender nonconforming necessarily desires medical or surgical interventions. However, medical gate-keepers drawing from Benjamin's research determined that only trans women both desiring medical intervention and expressing the wrong body diagnostics were approved for transition. This limited understanding of a trans body as somehow "wrong," as of trans women's bodies as somehow "male," continues to hold dominance over limitless alternative narratives of what it might feel like to be trans.

This necessity for such counter-narratives to this wrong body framework also continues to be manifested in contemporary cultural productions emerging from trans communities today. For example, Anna Anthropy's *Rise of the Video Game Zinesters* (2012) investigates DIY (do-it-yourself) video game production as a forum through which underrepresented subjects including trans women can demonstrate the narrative, medical, and cultural barriers set in place to constrict the movement of nonconforming bodies. As rule-governed spaces that urge players to consider relational and narrative constraints underlying the game's progression, the digital gaming format becomes an ideal arena to challenge the medicalization of trans identities and the impositions of medical access barriers attached to "wrong body" narratives. For instance, Anthropy's autobiographical videogame *dys4ia,* takes players through a labyrinth of consecutive "levels" of obstacles faced by trans people seeking access to transition. Upon entering "Level 2: Medical Bullshit," the game prompts players to "find a good clinic" that "doesn't force me to take a psych exam." Through its nostalgic 1980s retro-style graphics, the game presents a series of humorous but frustrating obstacles to accessing hormone therapy. To advance through the level, players must consider the cultural pertinence of the wrong body narrative and the barriers to access it creates. This second level, for instance, presents a playful clipboard containing a service-provider questionnaire complete with digitally presented medical questions that read:

Are you a woman?
Are you sure?
Are you really sure?
I don't believe you.

The player's avatar then is forced to fly literally through a series of hoops before arriving in a waiting room and moving through the nerve-wracking process of pathologization, assessment, diagnosis, and treatment access barriers that trans people must typically navigate. Through its imaginative, interactive format, the video game urges players to experience firsthand frustration with medical gatekeeping and to play with counter-narratives beyond the wrong body paradigm through which medical access might be granted.

These counter-definitions of trans identity such as Berry's understanding of his gender as "choirboy" can be positioned to contest this wrong body gatekeeping paradigm through which medical care for trans people is historically understood. Joanne Meyerowitz (2002, 130) traces the process by which the increasing availability of trans surgeries in the 1950s and 1960s was advanced not merely by clinical study but also by patient advocacy and persistent demands for access. Serano traces the adjacent history of medical research in the 1960s and 1970s that adopted Benjamin's publications and created even more rigorous gatekeeping barriers to surgery and hormone access. Serano (2007, 118) outlines that as trans people gained more attention in medicine and the media (all of it negative), the gatekeeping barriers that began to be standardized in the late 1960s further tightened the criteria necessary to qualify for transition. These rigid guidelines became the *Harry Benjamin International Gender Dysphoria Association (HBIGDA) Standards of Care* in 1979 that remained largely unchanged until the 1990s, mandating that in order to access transition, trans people had to (and even today, in most cases, still must) receive a DSM diagnosis of *Gender Identity Disorder*, now listed as *Gender Dysphoria* in the DSM-V (Serano 2007, 119).

Gaining access to this diagnosis, moreover, required trans women to present a narrative consistent with conceptions of femininity that were both gender-normative and heterosexual. Serano (2007) traces:

Most trans women understood that they needed to show up for their psychotherapy appointments wearing dresses and makeup, expressing stereotypically feminine mannerisms, insisting that they had always felt like women trapped inside men's bodies, that they'd identified as female since they were small children, that they were attracted to men but avoided intimate relations because they did not see themselves as homosexual, and that they were repulsed by their own penises. Those who did not follow this script risked having their requests for sex reassignment denied. (123-4)

Historically, women were only selected for transition if they had the financial resources to pay for therapy and medical care and only if their gender presentations prior to transition ensured they would be able to pass as female after transition (Serano 2007, 118-9). Serano illustrates the holdover of these beliefs into the current day, outlining that "such criteria ensured that cissexual prejudices about the preferred sizes and shapes of female and male bodies would be the ultimate arbiters of whether a trans person would be allowed to transition or not" (122). Such trends also reflect the medical agendas of mid-century sexological projects designed by the very same researchers to eradicate femininity in young boys and intersex infants, as trans gatekeeping was not an anomalous field of medicine but an extension of the medical trends to eliminate gender and sexual difference throughout the twentieth-century (119).

Speaking back to these historical biomedical practices in the present, *Choir Boy* accordingly demonstrates that trans subjects have always and continue to assert agency in opposition to gatekeeping barriers devised to erase their embodied differences. As their doctor-patient relationship develops, Berry attempts honest communication with his psychologist, using speech and not song to self-advocate for his need to access hormones. His provider's response defers back to biomedical authority, countering: "we can't prescribe without a clear diagnosis. GID is a diagnosis. 'Wants To Stay A Choirboy' doesn't show up in the DSM-IV" (187). This paradox rests in the fact that Berry's need to transition lies not in the wrongness of his body but in the rightness of his voice. Berry's experience is one that medical frameworks are unequipped to address on account of their rigid upholding of the Benjamin narrative by which they were formed. As Serano (2007) observes, the dominance of the wrong body narrative not merely shaped the way medical professionals view trans people but also shaped the way trans people "come to understand themselves" (116). Contesting the rigidity of DSM diagnostics and the medical professionals that enforce them not merely exhibits an individual act of resistance; Berry instead becomes an agent within the collective process of wrestling authority away from care providers and onto trans subjects as experts over their own access needs.

Consequently, Berry's ensuing gender transition (which begins illicitly without his doctor's awareness) likewise becomes incidental to his primary identification with his role in the choir. As Berry observes of the process, "to get the pills, even from the easy-going people at the Benjamin Clinic, you had to say you hated your body" (57). In making his gendered body secondary to its performative capacities, Berry moves the diagnostic narrative away from the body alone, hating not his body but only its capacity for pubescent vocal mutation, for granting him "a gift with an expiration date" (186).

Choir Boy, as a result, challenges the very narrative structure upon which the medicalization of trans identity rests. Just as trans scholars including Serano, Meyerowitz, and Stone identify the plurality of narratives that might exist if not for the inaugural and continued delineation of trans identity by medical gatekeepers, cultural texts by trans producers already offer a far more expansive range of tropes. As Serano (2007) reminds us:

> Those gatekeepers who believe that they alone should have the authority to determine who should and should not be allowed to transition ignore the obvious fact that gender dissonance has always been a 'self-diagnosed' condition: There are no visible signs or tests for it; only the trans person can feel and describe it. Once we make the arduous decision to transition—letting go of other people's perceptions of us in favor of being true to ourselves—there is really nothing anyone can do to stop us. For these reasons, medical and mental health professionals should turn their attention away from regulating sex reassignment and toward facilitating the safe access to the means of transitioning. (159-60)

Thus in contesting the limiting biomedical constructions of "trans," counter-fictions like *Choir Boy* intervene in this process of pathologization at the narrative level. As Susan Sontag (1978) observes, once bodies are medicalized, stigma gains influence upon people's own understandings of themselves, creating a form of social suffering that can only be confronted through an intervention within these very narratives.

Choirboys: a reality of the human condition

To better comprehend this process of reclaiming cultural scripts assigned to medicalized bodies, Berry's trans narrative can be placed in conversation with queer and feminist disability theory. Disability studies offers frameworks that position individuals with embodied differences as authorities over their own experiences, promoting self-advocacy and self-determination in relationship to medical care (Withers 2011, 36). Disability studies therefore provides a means of unpacking the culturally ingrained medical practices that locate trans-ness as something defined by service providers rather than something imagined with the narrative openness generated by trans people themselves. What disability studies can offer to de-pathologize trans bodies is multifold: disability theory locates non-normative bodies "as political, as valuable, as integral" (Kaefer 2013, 3). Disability studies also offers tools to reconcile trans patients' reliance on medical providers to meet their transition needs for surgeries and hormone therapies without framing their bodies as problems to be fixed or cured. In *Feminist Queer Crip* (2013), Alison Kaefer urges disability theory to pose complex questions about how to imagine futures that do not strive to eradicate disability but instead make space for ways of thinking and moving within the world that fail to adhere to normative gender and sexual embodiment (Kaefer 2013, 18; McRuer 2006, 9; Clare 1999, 111).

Tobin Siebers (2008), similarly, urges us to view different bodies not as problems but to instead regard "disability as a reality of the human condition" (6). Trans disability theorists including A.J. Withers also encourage a shift in focus from a medial model of fixing disabled bodies to a radical model of understanding how spatial, cultural, and social structures can be reworked to increase accessibility for all bodies that do not conform to a prescribed set of "healthy" norms (Withers 2012, 39; Kaefer 2013, 6). Siebers urges disability theorists to make space for complex questions of embodiment, pain, and medical intervention often overlooked by the social model of disability, without returning to the medical model's pathologizing of individual bodies as "defective" (Siebers 2008, 25; Kaefer 2013, 6). Rather than acting as gatekeepers who hold the discernment of whether to fix or cure wrong bodies, medical providers can work to support trans people's rights to self-determine their own embodiments, regardless of their gender identities or gender expressions (Serano 2007, 158). In juxtaposing the need for medical access with the understanding that not all bodies require or desire biomedical intervention, Siebers (2008) draws on disability studies to call for a theoretical model of "complex embodiment that values disability as a form of human variation" (25).

Echoing this very framework of human variation, Serano (2007) calls attention to the disservice of academics working from humanities perspectives that continue to pathologize trans subjects in manners parallel to that of clinical providers. Serano thereby raises critical concerns elemental to theorists working at the intersection of both. Serano argues:

> While researchers in the humanities often frame their work as being in opposition to that of the gatekeepers [. . .] the similarities between both groups far outweigh the differences. Both clinicians and academics are obsessed with meticulously documenting and subcategorizing the transgender population; both display the effemimanic compulsion of focusing primarily on MTF spectrum trans people; both view transsexuals as anomalies

that require explanation and justification rather than viewing us as a part of human diversity that just simply exists. (155-6)

Serano's call mirrors disability frameworks that view difference not as a problem to be solved but as an opportunity for medical providers to support individuals with embodied differences in attaining access to care. As Serano (2007) attests, this necessitates a shift from focusing on trans people as a problem and toward focusing on the reactions of cisgendered people *to* trans people as that which creates barriers to medical access (156). This mirrors the call of disability theorists to shift the focus away from disabled people and onto the systems that are disabling and that prevent accessibility medically and in all its intersectional forms. Regardless of how trans people fit into medical classifications of Gender Dysphoria, they should nevertheless have the right to self-identify with any gender they choose, and that gender should be seen as more legitimate than the one coercively assigned to them at birth (Serano 2007, 158).

Further, while much debate exists surrounding the classification of trans-ness as a disability or disorder (as trans activists dispute the utility of keeping Gender Dysphoria in the DSM versus removing it at the expense of individuals requiring insurance and access to care [Serano 2007, 160]), we must consider Douglas Baynton's (2001) historical analysis of groups wishing to remove themselves from categories of disability rather than fighting for the national inclusion of disabled people (31). While disability theorists including Bauman and Murray (2009) argue for the necessity to view disability and non-normative embodiments as valuable and positive, Siebers (2008) argues that disability has "both positive and negative valiances" and while disability as an *identity* should always be viewed as positive, we should also "resist the positive by acknowledging the negative—while never forgetting that its reason for being is to speak about, for, and with disabled people" (4,5). Siebers's assertion that disability is too complex to be considered in solely positive or negative terms connects to his argument that one can become disabled and suffer from pain and harmful social repercussions without holding any positive feelings about disability. Drawing on the example of an ableist white soldier who wakes up missing a limb, Siebers asks: "do people risk waking up one morning having become the persons whom they hated the day before. Imagine the white racist suddenly transformed into a black man, the anti-Semite into a Jew, the misogynist into a woman…" (26). In spite of the certainty with which Siebers poses this question, it can be argued that critical race studies and gender studies have already demonstrated how the culturally constructed lines between racial identities and genders are far less bounded than Siebers's analogy considers: all of us living in a white-supremacist, patriarchal, and ableist culture can easily internalize dominant beliefs regarding racism, misogyny, and disability even though these constructions of identity are just that and remain in constant flux. What *Choir Boy* suggests about both trans bodies in particular and difference in general is that until non-normative embodiments are regarded as positive and valuable within American culture, the onus will fall on those who are disabled to speak back to medical narratives that challenge their very right to exist.

Keep singing: vocal performance contesting pathology

Berry's challenge to this narrative process of medical gatekeeping rests in the power of his voice. In "Listening to Gender" (2007), Judith Ann Peraino identifies the salience of voice as a determinant of gender. Peraino explores how the performance of music, like the daily act of speech, can provide information regarding one's gender expression (64). Peraino considers the ways in which performers can offset an "alignment between voice and gender" through the discordance between one's voice and one's gender presentation. Peraino argues that while theoretically, "the aural component of gender operates as a secondary sex characteristic," the voice is actually "more primary in the determination of gender" (62). While the speaking voice, with its rigidly gendered expectations, might serve to limit the self-determination of one's gender expression, the singing voice, Peraino shows, can operate in boundless and performative ways, calling the signifying capacities of voice as a marker for gender into question. Trans cultural producers can accordingly play with vocal expectations to offset regulatory norms assigned to gender and identity. Vocal performance—the embodied rendering of sound—holds the power to affirm or to create discord with the gendering of the body from which the voice emerges. Through singing, yelling, and other limitless forms of noise-making that represents the bodies from which sounds emerge, vocal performance challenges essentialist understandings of gender upon which medical gatekeeping relies, opening up a space for trans subjects to self-determine their own gender expressions and access to medical care.

Berry's transition narrative subsequently rests not on conventional benchmarks of embodiment related to passing but on his desire to sing, to hit "that sweet spot choirboys struggle to reach" (117). When Berry attempts to castrate himself with a kitchen knife in his parents' house in order to preserve his vocal range (the act that lands him in the psychologist's office), his first thought after screaming and dropping the knife is of how "he'd hit that note, way up the windy scaffolding above everything, that nobody could reach at the end of Stanford's 'Te Deum' in C major" (42).

Much as vocal performance becomes the foundation of Berry's transition narrative, Berry survives persistent bullying, parental neglect, and self-harm by singing. Just as Peraino identifies the voice as a critical marker of gender and its performance, Berry's treble singing becomes a central facet of his gender identity and its expression. Berry's development, accordingly, is charted through an identification not with gendered signifiers but rather with musical ones. The novel opens with flashbacks to the inception of Berry's choir career, tracing:

> By the time the notes made sense to Berry, they had already claimed him on a level beneath reading and counting. He'd grasped the difference between a dotted quarter note (three quick leaps) and a triplet (three beats in two). He learned a thousand anthems by heart, but more than that, he understood something about the patterns of the music. You could count on music to change but return to its starting point, which made it more dependable than people. (4)

While most transition narratives focus on counter-normative identification with gendered behaviors, hairstyles, activities, or clothes, Berry's narrative complicates such tropes by linking the body and its gendering primarily with the body's ability to perform the language of music; Berry's performance of the notes becomes a stabilizing force more so than his gender, his peers, his teachers, or his unreliable parents. It is, accordingly, through vocal performance that Berry learns that "you can control every move your body makes but not your body itself" (35). The potential loss of control over his vocal performance threatens Berry with the "shatter[ing]" (36) of the stability he once found in the music. Berry experiences an acute sense of physical discomfort, suffering a "jagged clog" (36) in merely imagining the deepening of his voice. "The only thing I like about being a boy is the choir" (180), declares Berry, pointing to the capacities of musical performance in creating alternatives to the inevitable progression from (choir) boyhood to adult masculinity.

Parallel to the fictional Berry, trans musician Rae Spoon similarly plays with this gap between non-binary gender identification and the performance of voice. Like Berry's, Spoon's treble singing voice is central to Spoon's performance of their gender nonconforming identity. In the documentary *My Prairie Home* (2013), Spoon, in a moment of intimacy with the camera, ponders how "when you don't fit into the gender system, people tell you, 'you shouldn't exist, and you don't exist.'" Laughing, Spoon looks warmly into the camera and grinning announces, "I'm here to tell ya, I exist." *My Prairie Home,* as with the preceding works in Spoon's canon, sets up the listener to expect lower vocal ranges at critical moments within Spoon's performance wherein instead, Spoon raises their voice higher and higher, trilling out queer lyrics with choir boy sincerity. Singing in an octave that remains both incongruous with and central to Spoon's complex gender, the gap between vocal performance and vocal range becomes central to challenging the binary system of gender fundamental to gatekeeping medical diagnostics.

Alexis Mitchell's 2012 documentary, *The Break,* similarly asks viewers to consider the capacity of musical performance to challenge gender norms and gender-normative expressions of voice. Mitchell's film visually cuts together the moment of Justin Bieber's vocal transition at puberty to draw links between this pop icon and the experiences of trans musicians whose performances embody discrepancies between their genders and their vocal ranges. Reflecting on transition and vocal change, trans singer Alex Whyte shares in an interview for the film, "I've often thought if I could divide it up, and have it impact my speaking voice and not my singing voice, I'd prefer that." Whyte is framed intimately by the camera as he reflects on watching a moving vocal performance by the countertenor David DQ Lee. Whyte marvels that Lee's "tone was so pure, but really, really high. Later that night he was doing autographs and I [.. .] heard him speak, and his voice was super low [.. .] like a gruff man voice, and it just shocked me, it was so interesting, and yet, his singing voice, he sounded so comfortable there." In Mitchell's cinematic cutting together of theory (including the work of Peraino), interviews, performances, and popular culture, the film demonstrates that when musical capacity, rather than gender conformity, becomes a primary consideration within the process of gender transition, the medicalized limits assigned to narratives of gender embodiment must also necessarily shift.

Berry's desire to remain a choirboy, accordingly, requires access to medical care not because Berry holds a conventional wrong body narrative but because he is driven to safeguard against the deepening of his voice. Maura, who meets Berry in their therapist's waiting room, becomes a friend and mentor to Berry and teaches him how to access hormones as well as other survival tactics for being young and trans. Maura's experience as an adolescent sex worker speaks to the ways in which access to gender-confirming care intersects with access to employment. Maura and Berry find themselves dealing not merely with medical access barriers but other obstacles related to intersections between gender and class. Even Berry's engagement in singing reflects his class position, as Berry's initial involvement in the choir was motivated by the financial inaccessibility of other types of music lessons. While the choir offers Berry a skill set and a limited means of escape from his household, his own gender expression remains constricted through the barriers for class mobility that also constrain Berry's daily life. As Dean Spade (2011) identifies, "administrative policies and practices severely constrain access to health care and employment for most trans people" (12). Spade elaborates:

The most marginalized trans people experience more extreme vulnerability, in part because more aspects of their lives are directly controlled by legal and administrative systems of domination—prisons, welfare programs, foster care, drug treatment centers, homeless shelters, job training centers—that employ rigid gender binaries. (13)

Upon disclosing her profession to Berry, Maura reflects: "Seriously, I like my job. It's nice to be appreciated for being different, instead of hated. And I get to meet interesting people and fuck them" (167). Maura's experience therefore points to both the self-determination and economic empowerment of engaging in sex work and also to the institutional barriers Spade identifies that increase structural vulnerabilities to violence and criminalization.

These points of contact between structural access barriers and individual resiliencies in facing them also characterize Berry's experience of transitioning. As it changes, Berry's newly pubescent (and newly feminized) body becomes the site of violence but also of sexual pleasure: "with only cassock and surplice to cover them, Berry thought everybody must be able to see his buds [...] His music folder didn't cover anything. Everyone in church must be staring at Berry's chest. The thought sickened and thrilled him" (66). While Berry's trans body prompts violent reactions in his male and female peer groups alike, his chest also becomes eroticized by his girlfriend Lisa as the two exchange exploratory advances of intimacy and touch. Berry's chest also becomes valorized via its adornment in clothing, a pleasure Berry finds in garments from fashionable girls' dresses to ecclesiastic garb. While having his body change on hormones prompts Berry's experimentation with femme gender presentation and dress, his participation in the choir actually premeditates these moments of trans gender expression. A major highlight of choral performance for Berry is the requisite adornment in "cassocks and surplices." It is choirboy garments that initially grant Berry the pleasures of self-fashioning: "Berry never wanted to take his robe off. In regular clothes, he saw the rust that would swallow him eventually. But every time he caught his reflection in robes, he felt permanently stainless like the knife he wasn't thinking about" (51). Berry finds in the boys' choir something both masculine and treble, timeless and angelic, yielding the "intensifying pleasure ...[of] incandescent boys in their frocks" (63). Berry's transition also creates a sense of hyperawareness in his cassocks of his body as it changes. Berry refers to his growing chest as his "buds," a metaphor reflecting his desire upon transition to retain his choirboy identity as well as his given name: a choice to remain "Berry (like the fruit)" (305).

Berry's gender similarly aligns itself with musical expression and not binary biomedical conventions, eliciting his mother's frustration with her son's refusal to select a side of the gender binary. In so doing she too overlooks the significance of choral performance as a means of blending the two. "That's not an answer" (268), she retorts to Berry's gender identification as a choirboy, "You can't hide behind those robes forever. You need to make a commitment" (268). Because the choir is the foremost commitment in Berry's life, occupying hours of each day in rehearsal and the majority of Berry's fantasies and thoughts, his mother's imperative to "make a commitment" reflects the dictum that gender identification must override all else. When Berry's choral congregation and wider community later discovers that Berry is transitioning, organized pickets of the service take place, and Berry is nearly drowned by a vengeful Canon during a Baptism ritual. Faced with physical and public violence, it is the act of singing through which Berry asserts his own identity against the "angry people" (308) and for himself. Singing through the threats and the pain, Berry endures through the realization "that he could keep singing no matter what, no matter what anyone did to him. And that his voice could fill any space, no matter how big or awful, even into the dullest acoustics of despair and ear-blindness, he could keep singing" (308).

Berry's act of singing back to medical gatekeeping authorities offers imaginative opportunities for re-scripting imperatives that require all bodies conform to cultural sets of gendered and able-bodied norms. Anders's rendering of choirboy-as-gender-identity challenges medical service providers to shift from defining and limiting what constitutes a trans body toward facilitating access for everyone who requests medical or administrative intervention. Berry's determination to maintain the only part of boyhood he truly enjoys and to showcase a gender presentation expressed not through wrong body narratives but through his voice, motivates the revising of pathologizing trans narratives so that all bodies, like Berry's, could keep singing.

Acknowledgements I would like to thank Rebecca Garden and William Spurlin for all their editorial support and mentorship. I would also like to thank the editors at JOMH and all of the anonymous reviewers for their insights and feedback. This research was supported by the Social Sciences and Humanities Research Council of Canada.

References

Anders, Charlie. 2005. *Choir Boy*. Berkeley: Soft Skull.

Anthropy, Anna. 2011. *Dys4ia*. (Digital Game). Newground.

———. 2012. *The Rise of the Video Game Zinesters: How Freaks, Normals, Amateurs,Artists, Dreamers, Drop-outs, Queers, Housewives, and People Like You Are Taking Back an Art Form*. New York: Seven Stories.

Bauman, H-Dirkson L. and Joseph M. Murray. 2009. "Reframing: From Hearing Loss to Deaf Gain." *Deaf Studies Digital Journal* 1 (Fall): 1–10.

Baynton, Douglas. 2001. "Disability and the Justification of Inequality in American History." In *The New Disability History: American Perspectives*, edited by Paul K. Longmore and Lauri Umansky,: 33–57. New York: NYU Press.

Benjamin, Harry. 1954. "Transsexualism and Transvestism as Psychosomatic and Somatopsychic Syndromes." *American Journal of Psychotherapy*. 8 (2): 219–30.

———. 1966. *The Transsexual Phenomenon: A Scientific Report on Transsexualism and Sex Conversion in the Human Male and Female*. New York: Julian Press.

Clare, Eli. 1999. *Exile and Pride: Disability, Queerness, and Liberation*. Cambridge: South End.

Kaefer, Alison. 2013. *Feminist Queer Crip*. Bloomington: Indiana UP.

McMullen, Chelsea and Rae Spoon. 2013. *My Prairie Home*. Documentary. National Film Board of Canada.

McRuer, Robert. 2006. *Crip Theory: Cultural Signs of Queerness and Disability*. New York: NYU Press.

Meyerowitz, Joanne. 2002. *How Sex Changed: A History of Transsexuality in the United States*. Cambridge: Harvard UP.

Mitchell, Alexis. 2012. *The Break*. Film. Independent.

Peraino, Judith Ann. 2007. "Listening to Gender: A Response to Judith Halberstam." *Women & Music: A Journal of Gender and Culture* 11:59–64.

Serano, Julia. 2007. *Whipping Girl: A Transsexual Woman on Sexism and the Scapegoating of Femininity*. Emeryville: Seal Press.

Siebers, Tobin. 2008. *Disability Theory*. Ann Arbor: Michigan UP.

Sontag, Susan. 1978. *Illness as Metaphor*. New York: Farrar.

Spade, Dean. 2011. *Normal Life: Administrative Violence, Critical Trans Politics and the Limits of Law*. Cambridge: South End.

Stone, Sandy. 1991. "The Empire Strikes Back: A Posttransexual Manifesto." In *Body Guards: The Cultural Politics of Gender Ambiguity*, edited by Julia Epstein and Kristina Straub, 280–304. New York: Routledge.

Stryker, Susan. 2005. *Screaming Queens: The Riot at Compton's Cafeteria*. DVD. Frameline.

Withers, AJ. 2012. *Disability Politics & Theory*. Halifax: Fernwood.

Journal of Medical Humanities (2019) 40:33–51
https://doi.org/10.1007/s10912-018-9535-z

The Banality of Anal: Safer Sexual Erotics in the Gay Men's Health Crisis' *Safer Sex Comix* and Ex Aequo's *Alex et la vie d'après*

Jordana Greenblatt[1]

Published online: 17 August 2018
© Springer Science+Business Media, LLC, part of Springer Nature 2018

Abstract

Analyzing two harm reduction comics campaigns—one early in the AIDS crisis (the Gay Men's Health Crisis' [GMHC] 1980s *Safer Sex Comix*) and one more recent (Fabrice Neaud and Thierry Robberecht's 2008 *Alex et la vie d'après*), I explore tensions between queer safer sexual erotics and national discourses of sexual norms/deviation raised by Cindy Patton and William Haver at the height of AIDS discourse theory in 1996, approximately halfway between the comics. Using these theorists' reflections on the history of AIDS activism/representation as a hinge, I explore the manifestation/transformation a decade later of the ethical, educational, and erotic issues they raise. Both foreground the ways that HIV, safer sex, and/or eroticism pose difficulties for systems of linguistic and visual representation. Combining text and image, comics—a common harm reduction medium—epitomize this representational issue. While the GMHC addresses an immediate need for information about safer sex, *Alex* attempts to tackle the unrepresentability/unthinkability of safer and/or seropositive sex(uality). *Safer Sex Comix*, while largely prioritizing directness above formal experimentation, employ strategies of transgressing the borders of the comics panel to emphasize a plethora of lower-risk sexual acts. The most visually inventive moments in *Alex* represent Alex's feelings of unintelligbility post-diagnosis, but the comic restricts its representation of sex only to anal intercourse, and it proves unable to visualize alternative formulations of the erotic, turning to more normative narratives and images as earlier, visually explicit unsafe sexual encounters are replaced with more a/illusive representations post-conversion, literalizing the unrepresentability of seropositive erotic life.

Keywords HIV/AIDS · Graphic medicine · Safer sex · Educational comics · LGBTQ · Harm reduction

✉ Jordana Greenblatt
    jmgreenblatt@gmail.com

[1] Toronto, Canada

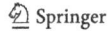

Facing the refusal of the US government to deal with the AIDS crisis, New York's Gay Men's Health Crisis began publishing *Safer Sex Comix* in the mid-1980s: sexually explicit harm reduction comics that represent lower risk sexual practices in image and text. Despite having received no federal funds, the comics were attacked by Jesse Helms (a right-wing US senator) in order to amend the 1987 AIDS appropriation bill to prohibit harm reduction material from benefiting from federal funding if it promoted same-sex sexual acts in any way. Just over two decades later, in 2008, Ex Aequo—whose organizational mandate is reducing transmission of HIV and other STIs among men who have sex with men (MSM) in Belgium's francophone community—published *Alex et la vie d'après*, by Fabrice Neaud and Thierry Robberecht. A longer comic,[1] *Alex* combines narrative, safer sex education, and strategies for constructing an erotic and relational life post-seroconversion. Sharing *Safer Sex Comix's* primary goal of transmission reduction among MSM, it received funding from a number of government sources. In comparing how texts at opposite historical edges of the genre (HIV harm-reduction comics published by non-government sexual health organizations serving MSM) depict sex, I draw from two canonical works of HIV/AIDS discourse theory: Cindy Patton's *Fatal Advice* and William Haver's *The Body of This Death*. Published in 1996, at the height of the *theoretical* genre (humanities and social science theorizations of the discursive and cultural position of HIV, informed by the then-new field of queer theory), they sit approximately halfway between the two comics campaigns. Extending the theorists' reflections on the history of AIDS activism and representation, I examine how the issues they raise shift, are reproduced, and/or resolved a decade later in the differing visual and textual vocabulary representing sex between men in the two comics campaigns. Beyond their cultural impact, available sexual vocabularies have potential epidemiological effects on the quality of sexual communication and the effectiveness of a given risk calculus. Aside from its role as a theoretical pivot-point, 1996 is key from a biomedical perspective; as Marsha Rosengarten points out, the introduction of HIV anti-retroviral combination drug therapy (ARVs) that year altered the way in which the embodied subject with HIV is materialized, a change that inevitably bears on the kinds of harm-reduction material I consider.[2]

In negotiating between two key HIV/AIDS discourse theorists at the height of their discipline and two harm reduction campaigns that temporally bracket it, I explore the contradictions that emerge in tensions between envisioning queer safer sexual erotics and national discourses of sexual norms and deviation. Both *Safer Sex Comix* and *Alex et la vie d'après* intersect with concerns raised by Patton and Haver in ways that develop with and are necessarily conditioned by their historical contexts. Neither work can possibly represent all MSM-directed safer-sex comics campaigns of its era—either in the West or in its national context—but they both still express their relationships to national idea(l)s of the citizen, flagged conspicuously by the (un)availability of government funding, in characteristic ways. While, for example, *Safer Sex Comix* lack the comedic tone of the German organization Deutsch AIDS-Hilfe's *Safer Sex Comic* campaign of the same era, both express the sexual riotousness prevalent in queer campaigns lacking government support. Meanwhile, while *Alex*'s native Belgium hardly possesses a uniform national identity given the often-heated divisions between its Dutch- and French-speaking communities, as an organization serving and funded by Belgium's francophone regions and populations, Ex Aequo's project is defined by national(ist) categories. National(ist) propensities are evident, for example, in its efforts to include members of immigrant communities such as Rachid by presenting them as no different than any other franco-phone character—and thus possessing no distinct concerns. As the seat of the EU's headquarters, Belgium also performs a central role in grounding a broader, shared European citizen-identity.

Sexual citizenship is central to Western national ideals in ways that exceed European/North American divisions. Carl Stychin's work on law, citizenship, and sexuality, for example, indicates that, while details vary, both European and North American norms of sexual citizenship circulate around heteronormative ideas of sex and family.[3] Patton investigates establishments of sexual divisions that define national norms through educational strategies, which often occlude or deeroticize safer sex practices indigenous to queer erotic cultures. Since available representations of how to *practice* safer sex necessarily also select which sex acts they address, safer sex campaigns define what counts, or should count, as sex through their very omissions—often, omissions of low risk acts indigenous to queer cultures that are not heteronormatively legible as sex itself. Meanwhile, Haver suggests that dominant HIV/AIDS discourses avoid ways in which thinking AIDS presses us to imagine the erotic at the edge of the thinkable. Because HIV threatens our normative idea(l)s of the bounded, discrete body, erotic practices that rely less on such ideas—which Haver frames as productively perverse— may also be more productive when it comes to safer sex and to envisioning seropositive bodies as functionally erotic. Nevertheless, neither the erotic nor HIV are representationally straight-forward, and both Haver and Patton foreground the ways that HIV, safer sex, and/or eroticism pose difficulties for systems of linguistic and visual representation.

In combining text and image, comics, an extremely common harm reduction medium, combine and mitigate these difficulties. While *Safer Sex Comix* address a more immediate (and episodic) concern with informing about safer sex at a time when envisioning a functional subjectivity for living long-term with HIV was hardly a relevant concern, *Alex* begins to tackle the unrepresentability or unthinkability of safer and/or seropositive sex(uality). The most visually inventive moments in *Alex* represent Alex's feelings of unintelligibility post-diagnosis: a sense of bodily upheaval that does not lend itself easily to literal representation. But the comic is ultimately unable to visualize alternative formulations of the erotic, turning instead to more conventional narratives and images as earlier, visually explicit unsafe sexual encounters are replaced with more allusive and illusive encounters post-conversion, literalizing the unrepresentability of seropositive erotic life and desire/desirability. In *Alex*, the *only* sex is anal intercourse, and even that is no longer graphically depicted by its conclusion, where it is largely replaced by kissing and cuddling. A gulf, then, exists between (or beside) the acts representable in *Alex*, which are the ones most clearly legible (as definitely sex and definitely not) to a heteronormative eye. The plenitude of sexual acts represented in *Safer Sex Comix* vanishes into the specificity of one sex act that comes to function as "sex" itself in *Alex*.

And, indeed, both Patton and Haver comment on discursive practices arising in response to the AIDS crisis that narrow a diversity of sexual acts or narratives into one act that becomes definitional of "gay sex" and of gay male identity itself. As Patton notes, over time, both the national discourse and queer safer sex campaigns positioned penetrative vaginal or anal intercourse as "sex" itself (1996, see 76, 106-7), an observation now so mainstream that it appears in Dan Savage's advice column. "The persistent focus on condoms and their associ-ation with the new gay male sexuality of the AIDS era," Patton writes, "... insisted that intercourse, the riskiest practice, was to be the mature and stable form of homosexual sex, the ideologically 'safe' deviation" (1996, 76). As Gary Dowsett notes in a more recent study, "we can never know whether an increased interest in the practice of anal sex between men is a consequence of the densities of association made possible by the development of modern gay communities or by the emphasis placed upon that practice over the past 25 years of HIV prevention, or both" (2009, 231). However, regardless of whether this increase is the *result* of the educational emphasis placed on anal sex, such framings of "sex" have continued, in the time since Patton's concerns were published, to discursively marginalize other sexual practices, ones that are, indeed, less epidemiologically risky.

From a cultural, erotic, and theoretical standpoint, this occlusion represents a significant loss, curtailing a creative plenitude of erotic acts and enjoyment in favor of more strictly defined and definable categories. From an epidemiological one, it can, at the very least, result in confusion about the relative risk levels of the varied sex acts that fall outside the category of penile-anal intercourse, which can reduce the effectiveness of a given risk calculus. These two standpoints of loss affect and complicate each other. When "sex" becomes discursively delimited as but one thing, other acts that fall outside of its purview—even ones that have historically been considered and enjoyed as "sex" within queer erotic cultures—can be assumed to be insufficient *as* a sexual encounter. In other words, assumed insufficient in the very situations in which to so assume is most epidemiologically and erotically counterproductive. Particularly in interactions involving younger people, who may not yet have developed their skills in communicating and negotiating their desires, such discourses can result in both parties assuming that the other party must desire a certain act, given the implication that everyone does, even when neither party does and both are more effectively erotically fulfilled by other things.[4] While increased understanding of the vast landscape of sexual tastes and ability to communicate one's desires is part of growing and aging, the discursive availability of a range of activities as "sex itself" at a given age can help to broaden what *can* be communicated in sexual interactions, an effect that serves the ends both of risk negotiation and sexual enjoyment.

All of this, of course, is not to say that there are not many people who do or should enjoy and want to have anal sex, nor is it to say that information about how to have it more safely is not crucially important. Nor, indeed, is it to say that people are no longer having other kinds of sex. However, the exclusion of alternatives from the discursive category of sex can result in encounters that increase risk, while sometimes simultaneously decreasing erotic fulfillment. As risk management suffers in the discursive narrowing of "sex," the erotic also loses, both practically and conceptually. Indeed, Haver, like Patton, laments the occlusion of the perverse, presenting perversity as both philosophically and politically crucial. For him, the perverse's ability to envision the erotic outside even of "a narrative of teleological orgasm" is where it is at its most philosophically and ethico-politically interesting (1996, 153). To different degrees, both Patton and Haver represent the narrowing of what constitutes "sex" as an erotic attrition that, aside from its more esoteric negative philosophical effects, also has the practical result of discursively marginalizing queer sexual practices that effectively balance concerns of safety and excitement from broader conversations.

The restrictive definition of sex and the emphasis on reasserting the body as discretely contained that emerges from this discursive practice (potentially intersecting with differential degrees to which queer sexual subjects are treated as inside or outside the national body, expressed through the availability of public funds) leads to the functional unrepresentability of seropositive erotic bodies by the end of *Alex*. While policies such as Helms' aforementioned amendment deny marginal sexual populations public resources, they thereby leave defining queer sex in the hands of queer people themselves. Policies that include queer subjects as citizens, via funding and other means, still generally define the national subject through the lens of the (hetero) *normative* subject and implicitly encourage marginal communities to define themselves analogously—a definition that tends to exclude the perverse and the culturally specific.

If we bring Haver's and Patton's arguments into conversation, we can synthesize a theory of the perverse as that which is, at once, culturally specific, never fully representable in language or image, and replete with acts that are both low risk epidemiologically and indefatigably erotic. Safer-sex comics campaigns have the option to push the limits of erotic representability, emphasizing a range of possible practices and pleasures or to narrow and solidify the limits of representable sex. According to Patton, the latter strategy affects even colloquial sexual language, explaining, "Even the term fucking—once a term for a wide range of connotations—became the unified term for penile-anal or penile-vaginal intercourse, that is, for the potentially 'bad' thing" (1996, 114). As Patton observes, sexual cultures have complex structures of communication and acts—ones that are not always translatable into the dominant discourse. Describing her involvement with a late 80s safer sex project, Patton claims that its goal, "unlike efforts to 'eroticize' safe sex, [was to] retrieve already and always safe activities like jerking off, licking, tit-play, verbal scenes, etc., not by proposing them as substitutes, but by returning them to their former status as core elements of queer erotic life" (1996, 124). This goal was in opposition to campaigns that "ultimately situated penile-anal intercourse as the most important form of sex, even if only as that which was lost and must now be mourned. Licking, rubbing, watching, fantasizing—the very practices that were once considered fetishistically absorbing and gratifying, and still the safest practices from the standpoint of HIV transmission—were tacitly reduced to poor substitutes, foreplay, or occasions for discussing the safety of practices to be engaged in later" (106).

As we will soon see, by the time we get to *Alex*, these practices have disappeared even *as* substitutes, foreplay, or the occasion for discussion from both the linguistic and visual landscapes. While readers' *use* of pornographic comics in their capacity as masturbatory aid may necessarily recuperate some of Patton's vanishing queer practices, the premise of safer sex pornography—that readers will reproduce, in their multi-person sex, the practices that they have learned about in their masturbatory material—indicates a clear limit to which practices *Alex* is able to envision beyond the solitary act. The degree to which "sex" narrows in its pages suggests that earlier efforts to combat the normative citizen-focused pedagogy's discursive narrowing of "sex" through shifting how sex is figured in harm reduction educational material were neither unwarranted nor sufficiently successful. *Alex*'s ability to deal sensitively with the difficulties of achieving a functional post-diagnosis sense of self stems, in part, from the project's basis in interviews with HIV-positive men. However, its own difficulty with representing sexual pleasure—and its diversity—especially when it comes to seropositive bodies, suggests that questions about suffering may have outweighed questions about pleasure in the project's conceptualization, an oversight that may hinder the goals both of alleviating suffering and of reducing transmission. Though *Alex*'s interviewees are drawn from Ex Aequo's national and linguistic target population, their answers express infection histories and long-term anxieties consistent with common North American narratives. Meanwhile, the failure of the interview excerpts to address pleasure and the comic's emphasis on relinquishing casual encounters in favor of implied monogamy echo criticisms of "gay promiscuity" within assimilationist American gay culture. Douglas Crimp (1987) objects to such criticisms using mainstream-successful work by Randy Shilts and Larry Kramer[5] as examples, and similar normativizing discourses reemerge in recent criticisms of pre-exposure prophylaxis (PrEP) by mainstream American gay figures such as Dan Savage, Zachary Quinto, and, again, Kramer.[6] As Crimp puts it, framing activities going on in gay bathhouses as "unimaginable" is "a way of saying that certain sexual acts are beyond the pale for most people," a discursive strategy that resonates with the representational limitations of *Alex* (1987, 244).

To return to Patton and Haver, Patton's argument is, of course, much more practical than Haver's unapologetically high theory approach. Nevertheless, her emphasis on the political and cultural value of perverse eroticism not as a substitute for "sex" but *for its own sake* intersects with the more abstract considerations of Haver's work. Patton concludes her monograph with the suggestion that

> The next step may be … to reject any idea of a wholesome "gay lifestyle." Instead, we must think about sex as the form of power that makes and saves queer lives. This requires us to stop defining and promoting an object, *a* sex that can be categorically distinguished from its multiple Others, the ones that are sustained as dangerous, deadly, etc. There is only *one* dangerous act, being fucked without a condom, the sole act, not coincidentally, which is evoked by the national pedagogy as the citizen's "freedom" … (1996, 155, emphasis hers)

The "free" citizen is the citizen so normative, so comfortably regarded as low risk *at the level of identity* (i.e. straight, white, purportedly monogamous, non-drug using, etc.), that they can have easily-heteronormatively-recognizable sex without condoms, without much fear or judgment, regardless of actual risk-level. Conversely, the national pedagogy establishes the perversely erotic—largely acts with low or no risk of transmission—as dangerously unthinkable. Dangerous, that is, because they threaten what Haver, drawing from David Wojnarowicz, refers to as the One Tribe Nation—the nation of the citizen whose sociality excludes the erotically perverse even from the realm of the other deserving compassion. While the One Tribe Nation that Haver discusses is the US, *Alex* espouses similar values of wholesomeness, given its positioning of implied monogamy as happy ending.

For Haver, the AIDS crisis, the AIDS object, and the question of the erotic can, at their discursive best, push us towards the edges of the philosophically and erotically thinkable. They offer "the ultimately unspeakable radical historicity and sociality of erotic existentiality. … the 'body of this death,' the erotic body in its historicity and sociality, an unimaginable figure, designates the thought of that which it is ultimately impossible to think" (1996, xi). In other words, both AIDS and the erotic press us to consider the uncontainable abundance and creativity of historically and socially contingent sexual cultures and subjectivities. This crisis of figurability emerges most relevantly in the harm reduction material I will come to shortly in both the perverse that is not reducible to *a* sex and the disappearance of the erotic seropositive body that is such a crisis of figurability's partial effect. Ultimately, Haver's "conjunction of the ethical, the political, and the perverse … a politics of inconsolable perversity" (xvi) appears only as lack in the later of the two comics. This failure of figuration stems from and supports the reassertion of "clean and proper … bodies," which removes the erotic from epistemic availability, as "as long as the erotic is conceived to be a simple transaction … between an unproblematic self and a disgusting but nonetheless essentially unproblematic other … then HIV transmission can only be conceived in terms of the instrumentality of the body … But this is to attempt in a certain prophylaxis to occlude the erotic altogether, which is in the same occlusion to attempt a prophylaxis against historicity and sociality" (12). Now, Haver never suggests that the erotic is reducible *only* to sex; however, the intersection of the two *is* the dominant concern of safer sex harm reduction comics.

Safer Sex Comix are short, instrumental, serial, and, as result, not terribly formally experimental—although it is worth noting that they regularly transgress the edge of the comics panel with images of cocks, balls, come shots, and a leather daddy's pants: perverse sexuality, or at least perverse sexual functions, as, for example, the leatherboy in Issue 5 (Fig. 1) neither orgasms nor wants to, while the leather daddy's cock is initially most interesting for its ability to piss rather than to ejaculate, and come shots in each issue do not function as a coda to penetration because no penetration takes place. The comics represent a variety of already culturally present safer sexual acts as highly erotic, usually without drawing attention to them as "other" than the rest of sex, although *Safer Sex Comix #2* does address safer sex malaise, beginning with a character stating: "I'm pissed off ... sex isn't fun anymore!!" (Greg and Bodenschatz 1986).[7] *Safer Sex Comix* represent a plenitude of graphic depictions of longstanding sexual practices and sites of fetishistic pleasure within a variety of erotic subcultures. Specifically, the come shot—and except in an issue depicting phone sex, ejaculating *on* another man's body—is a feature of every issue to which I have access. *Safer Sex Comix #5: Leatherman* (Fig. 1), for example, does not mourn lost sex, depicting instead a series of acts native to leather culture that have traditionally often been sufficient *as* sex, specifically golden showers and, inevitably in this series, ejaculating on someone else.

Of course, the come shot is a mainstay of pornographic representation of male sexuality, which makes its presence in *Safer Sex Comix*, which I will return to in more depth after elucidating the sexual dynamics and elisions of *Alex*, seem to go without saying and its notable absence from *Alex* even more curious. I do argue that there is one come shot in the later comic (Fig. 2), but the visual metaphor is so closely conflated with one of detumescence that, coming when it does, it serves only to reify the unthinkablity of the erotic seropositive body, particularly its fluids. Alex, newly returned to sex after a long hiatus, begins a relationship with Michel but decides not to reveal his seropositive status until he knows that their relationship will last. Michel arrives with a bottle of champagne to celebrate their one month anniversary, only to have Alex disclose his HIV status as the cork pops. After a stunned moment, Michel says "mais tu m'a rien dit"—"but you told me nothing"—over an image of the tiny, penis shaped cork falling to the ground (Robberecht and Neaud 2008, 36).[8] Now, of course, Alex's lack of disclosure is experienced as an extreme violation, but the image of near simultaneous orgasm and detumescence also reflects the ongoing status of the seropositive body in this narrative.

The failure to explore the desire and desirability of seropositive bodies in *Alex* comes as a surprise, given the comic's attention to Alex's subjective re-construction elsewhere. In other ways, the thinkability of the seropositive body is much more explicitly (and creatively) dealt with. A large part of *Alex* focuses on his process of achieving a workable self-perception and being-in-the-world post-diagnosis. The very title of the comic—*Alex et la vie d'après*, or Alex and the life afterwards—echoes Haver's observation that AIDS narrative is often constellated around "the problematization of the very categories of 'inside' and 'outside'; or the establishment of 'the diagnosis' as the barrier that henceforth divides a pre-test 'before' ... from the horrors of the unavoidable ever-after" (1996, 125). The most visually creative moments of *Alex* take place against the edge of the thinkable of the self—the HIV positive self. We see this creativity in the depiction of Alex adjusting to his medication, which begins visually psychedelic and includes an image of him riding his pillbox (Fig. 3). Robberecht and Neaud depict the disruption of inside/outside containment boundaries in Alex's vision of himself as a monster spewing viruses, shouting: "Fuyez tous!! Je suis le grand contaminateur!"—"Flee, everyone!! I am the great contaminator" (Fig. 4). These visually creative moments extend to Alex's inability to self-perceive as an erotic body, implying a promise to seek out the edge of the perversely erotically thinkable that is never fulfilled. In visualizing his own lack of desire,

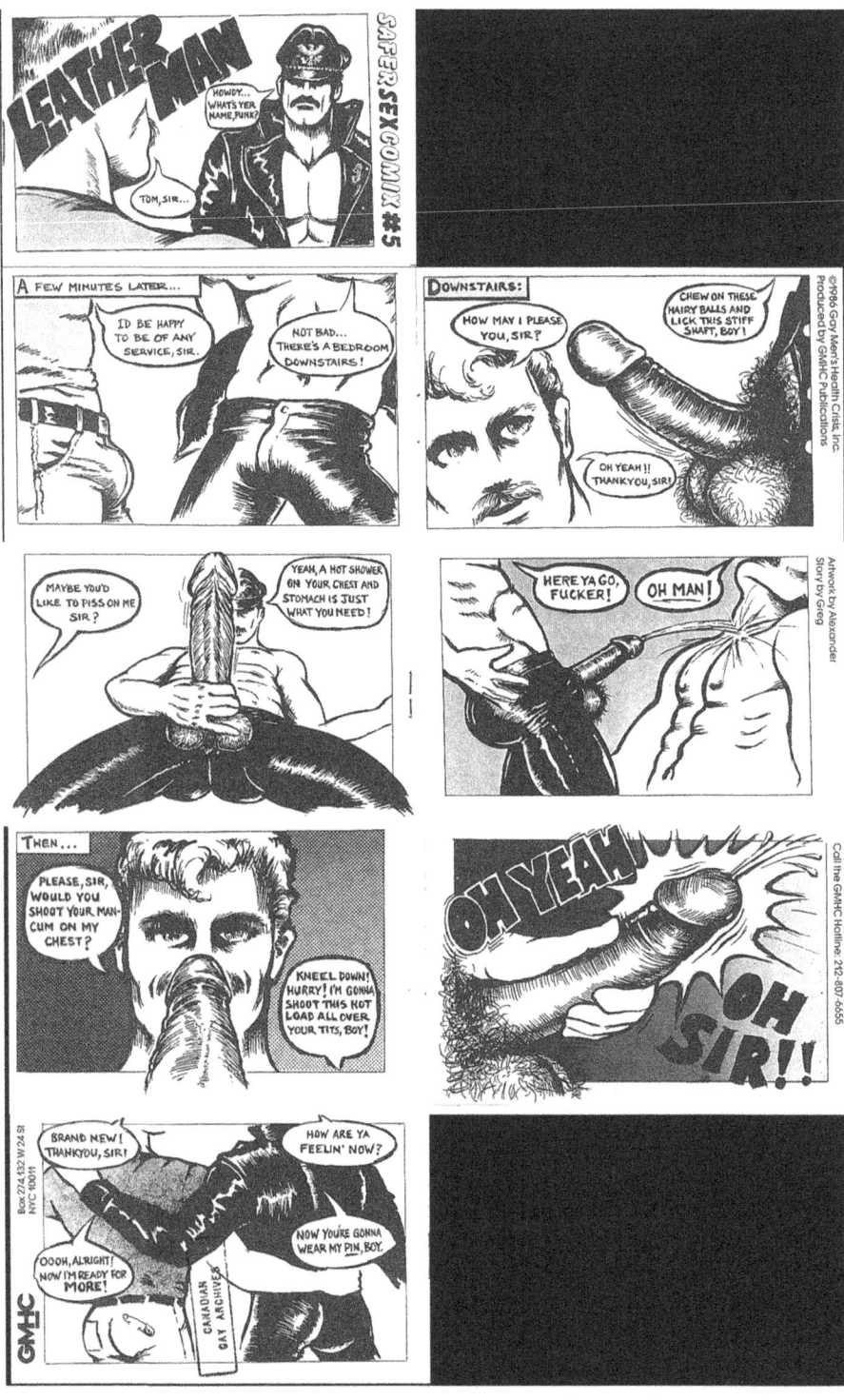

◀ **Fig. 1** *Safer Sex Comix #5: Leatherman*, which represents an interaction between a leather daddy and a submissive "boy" including piss play and ejaculation on the submissive partner, is reproduced here in its entirety. (Story by Greg and artwork by Alexander. *Safer Sex Comix #5: Leatherman*. [New York: GMHC Publications, 1986]. Courtesy of Gay Men's Health Crisis, New York)

he imagines his body with Xs over his head and crotch (Robberecht and Neaud 2008, 15). And, when he is rejected in a bar after revealing his HIV status, he visualizes himself wearing a sign around his neck that reads "séropo" (seropositive), standing alone on a blurred dark patch on an otherwise white floor, surrounded by staring men (21). Finally, when Michel leaves him, his bodily boundaries seem literally to disintegrate (Fig. 5).

Clearly, *Alex* must negotiate a set of concerns that were not yet relevant at the time in which *Safer Sex Comix* were produced: how to live long-term with HIV. As Rosengarten asserts (albeit with the important qualifier that not all—or even most—HIV-positive people have access to treatment), "it is possible to claim that as a result of ARVs, HIV and AIDS have

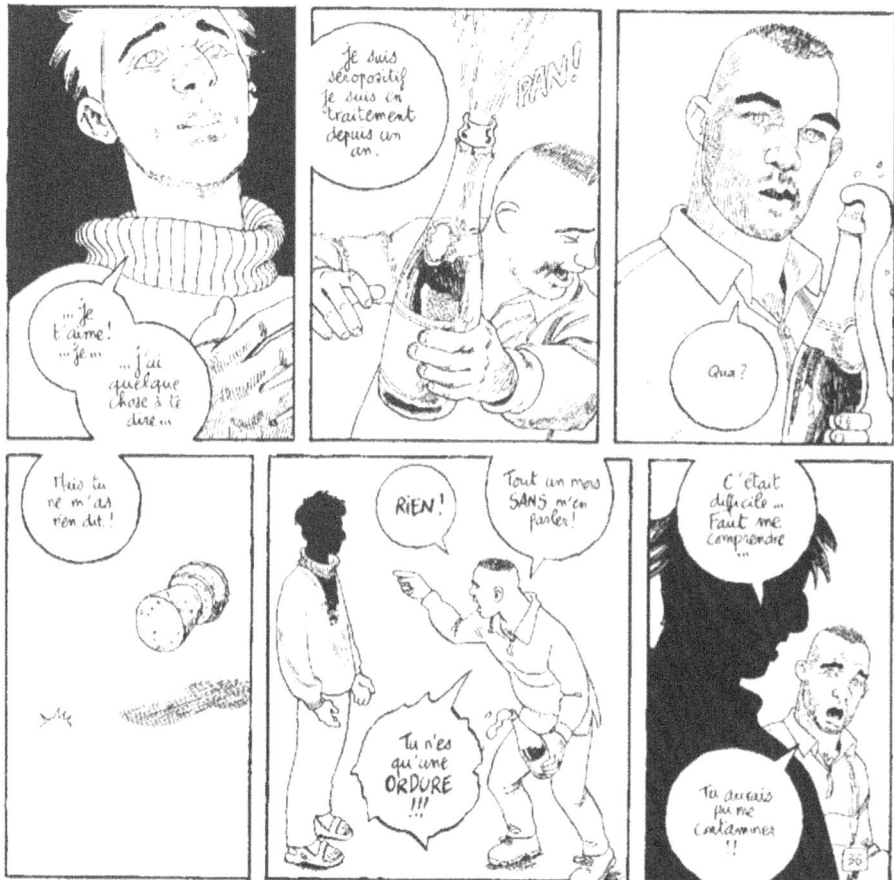

Fig. 2 Michel celebrates his and Alex's one-month anniversary with an ejaculatory spray of champagne, only to hear Alex's disclosure of his HIV-positive status as the cork falls to the floor. (Story by Thierry Robberecht and artwork by Fabrice Neaud. *Alex et la vie d'après*. [Brussels: Ex Aequo, 2008], 36. Courtesy of Ex Aequo, Brussels)

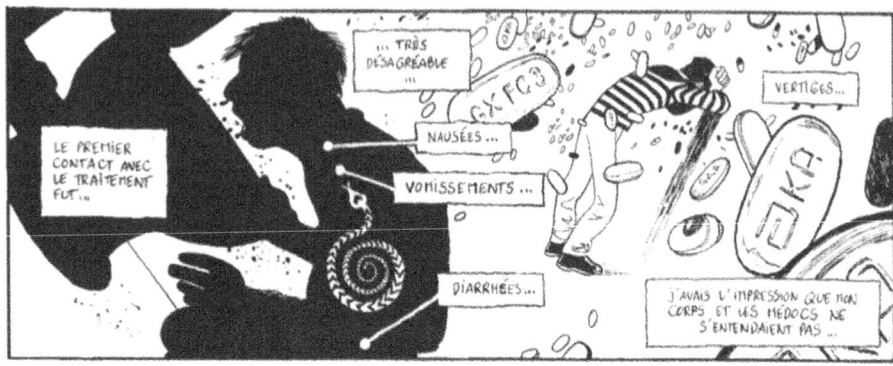

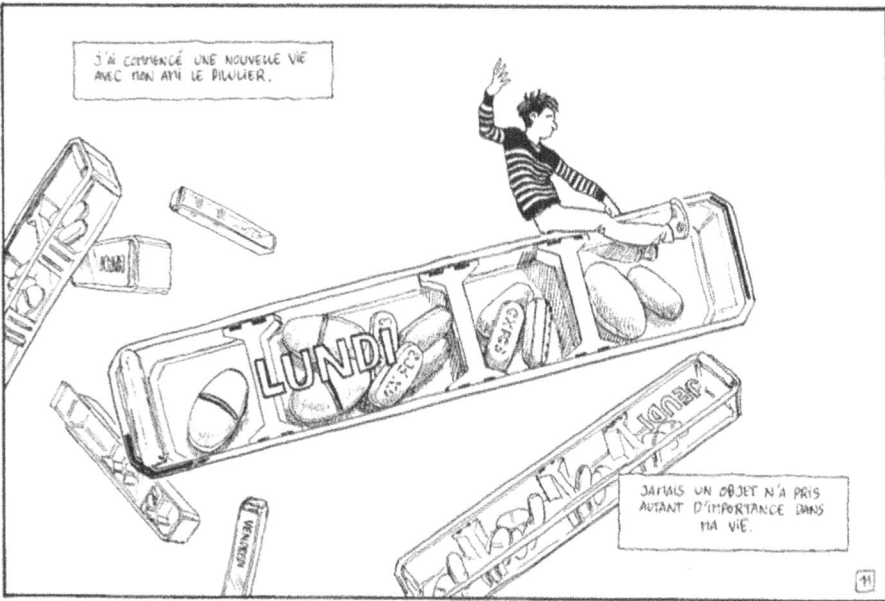

Fig. 3 Psychedelic representation of Alex's adjustment to his medication's negative side-effects, followed by a depiction of Alex riding his pillbox through a blank background. (Robberecht and Neaud. *Alex*, 11. Courtesy of Ex Aequo, Brussels)

become 'decoupled,' so to speak" (2009, 3). This decoupling results in a need for material supporting the long-term subjectification strategies of newly HIV-positive people that exists alongside the need for transmission-prevention campaigns and strategies. *Alex* strives to do both. As Rosengarten attests (as, in less theoretical language, do Ex Aequo's interviewees), "the terrain of treating and living with HIV remains, for many, immensely complicated and distressing" (4). Functionally, given the shift in HIV-positive longevity, one of the major changes that takes place in 1996 regarding HIV/AIDS is one of temporality, and temporality itself is central to Alex's narrative of adjustment—his process of navigating a newly complicated and distressing terrain.

The division between, as Haver terms them, the pre-test before and the ever-after is present in *Alex* but in a manner that temporarily destabilizes its temporal linearity. Alex's reaction to his initial diagnosis, "Je crois que je peux toucher du doit l'instant ou j'ai été infecté"—"I believe that, with my finger, I can touch the instant in which I was infected," seems to suggest

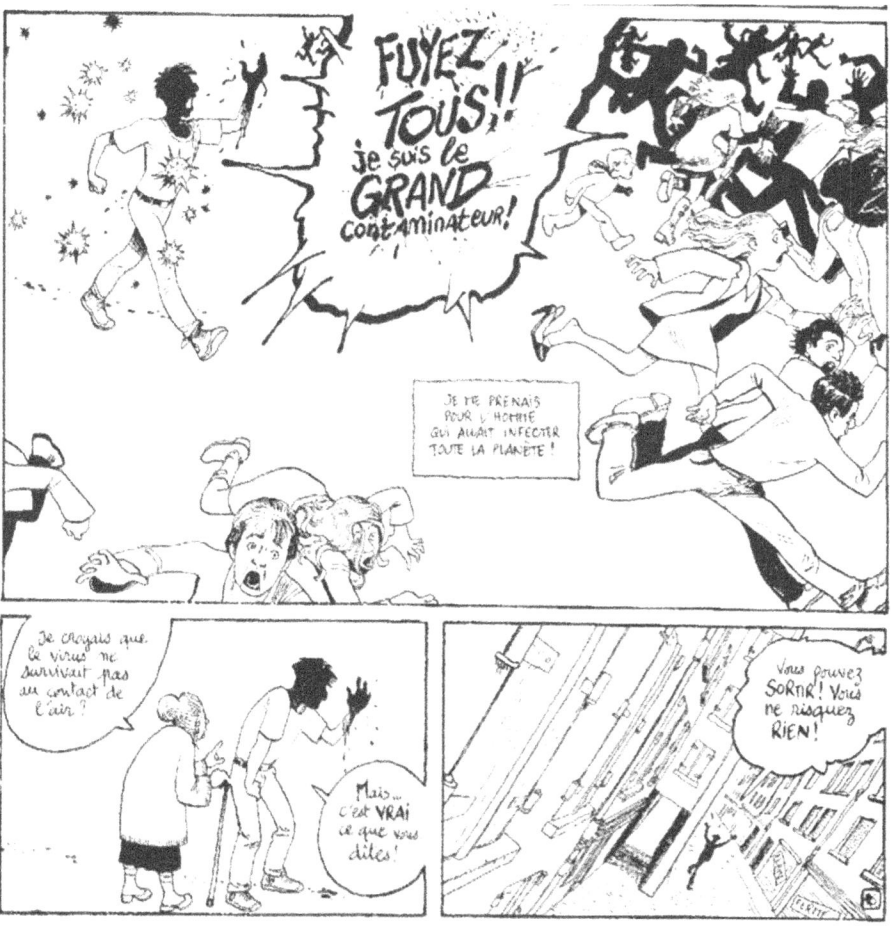

Fig. 4 Alex envisions himself as a monster spewing viruses after cutting himself while chopping onions. (Robberecht and Neaud, *Alex*, 16. Courtesy of Ex Aequo, Brussels)

temporal fixity and a firm dividing line between before and after (Robberecht and Neaud 2008, 2). However, the visual landscape destabilizes temporality in the moment of diagnosis, as Alex, in his chair, and his doctor, behind her desk, lift up and float apart in the suddenly blank emptiness that had been the doctor's office, and Alex leaves the doctor behind to return to his moment of infection. As Alex begins medication, Robberecht and Neaud's treatment of his adjustment period emphasizes not only the inextricability of body, self, and biotechnology that Rosengarten describes throughout her oeuvre but also their intimate relationship to temporality. Alex experiences the side effects of his medications against the same white, vacant backdrop he experiences immediately after diagnosis (Fig. 3). As Rosengarten details, the side-effects of HIV medication are not only physical but include the temporal effect of "the almost unmanageable nature of dosing regimens that can require taking up to seven pills three times a day and at different specified periods, before food, with food, and after food" (2009, 19). Neaud's drawing of Alex riding his pillbox through the blank, white background effectively brings together Alex's medical regime's hyper-regimentation of his temporality and its participation in the temporal disorientation of his newly experienced bodily

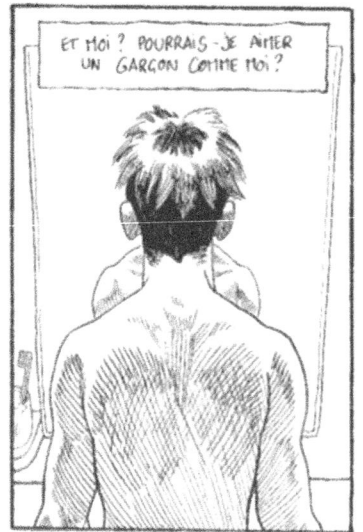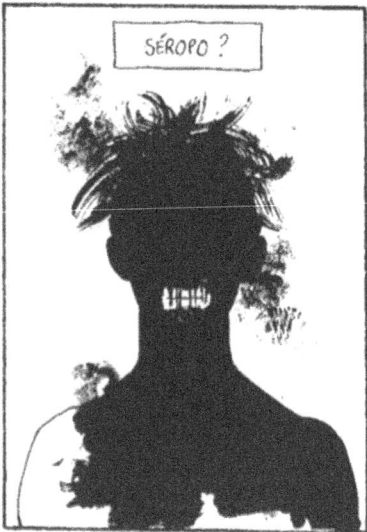

Fig. 5 Alex envisions his face in the mirror as an outlineless, featureless, dark blur after being rejected by Michel. (Robberecht and Neaud. *Alex*, 38. Courtesy of Ex Aequo, Brussels)

disorderliness, which refuses to adhere to orderly models of the outside word—including normative temporalities (Fig. 3). As Alex observes, "J'ai commencé une nouvelle vie avec mon ami le pilulier. Jamais un object n'a pris autant d'importance dans ma vie"—"I started a new life with my friend the pillbox. Never had an object taken on so much importance in my life" (Robberecht and Neaud 2008, 11). Biomedicine, in the form of the pillbox, both organizes and destabilizes Alex as an HIV-positive body and subject.

Or, at least, attempted subject, because much of what is destabilized in Alex's earlier attempts to negotiate his being-in-the-world post-diagnosis revolves around a destabilization of self and of bodily containment boundaries. Alex's fantasy of himself as a monster spewing viruses after he cuts his finger cutting onions is part of an ongoing disruption of the self as a discrete body throughout *Alex,* at least at its best (Fig. 4). His vision of his own face as an outlineless, featureless blur after being rejected by Michel similarly suggests that the disruption of his bodily and subjective containment boundaries are an integral part of his struggle, very much in keeping with Haver's observation about the centrality of the disruption of inside/outside categories to AIDS narrative (Fig. 5). However, rather than build new models of self and of self/other relationships to build new subjects, temporalities, and pleasures—in erotically and epidemiologically productive ways—*Alex* tends to reassert conventional structures and boundaries of the self, relationships, and temporality, ones much in keeping with the values of the citizen or at least those "deserving" the citizen's compassion in its effort to offer a model for long-term, HIV-positive life.

Ultimately, the resistance to the erotically perverse—the erotically varied—expressed in *Alex* is complicit with the occlusion of the erotic seropositive body that occurs by the story's end, despite earlier promise that the work is trying to imagine the borders of the HIV positive self and the erotic at their point of intersection. Alex eventually loses the metaphorical Xs over his head and crotch, regaining his sexual desire for other people, but neither his own sexual enjoyment nor the prospective desirability of seropositive bodies are ever effectively visualized. This absence is a significant loss. As Rosengarten observes, "Sex can be understood as a remarkably enduring and changing feature of the epidemic: not only as a source of transmission but also as a source of the most conceptually and materially effective intervention" (2009, 63). And, in *Alex*, unlike in *Safer Sex Comix*, sex truly is only one thing. There are kissing and cuddling, which are definitely not sex, and intercourse, which definitely is. Nothing else. Now, this is not surprising when it comes to the stories of seroconversion at the comic's outset, but it becomes increasingly troubling later.

Indeed, sex of any kind seems less and less thinkable or visualizable as the narrative proceeds. Initially, the scenes of seroconversion are quite graphic, except for Rachid's.[9] Alex's scene of infection involves a close-up drawing of his sex partner's erect penis, as well as a soft-core drawing of anal intercourse, with Alex as the penetrative partner.[10] Gilles' involves a very graphic drawing from below of anal penetration. Both Alex and Gilles locate their moments of infection in casual encounters. Rachid, however, is infected by a man with whom he lived for six months, who never disclosed his status, and the visual representation of Rachid having sex with his ex is discreet, with Rachid recognizably drawn and his partner nothing but a dark silhouette. This last representation is the first indication of the text's tendency to be unable to represent love (even one sided, as in this case) and sex in the same moment.

As *Alex* progresses, sex becomes less and less explicit and less and less represented. When Alex meets Vincent, also seropositive and Alex's first sexual partner after his diagnosis, the sex they have can be seen in Fig. 6. Now, contextually, it is clear what is happening, but I argue that this scene is not as explicit, even, as the soft-core depiction of Alex's moment of infection, which we can see by comparing Alex's sex with Vincent to an equivalent image from *Safer Sex Comix #1*, which, despite its visual similarity to Alex's sex with Vincent, actively informs the reader that penetration is *not* happening. One of the characters states, "Shit coach … that stiff dick of yours feels so fucking good sliding *against* my ass" (Fig. 6, emphasis mine). The image in *Alex*, then, is both vague *and* specific—specific only because we know that there is only *one* sex act in this comic. Alex's sex with Michel is even more allusive (Fig. 7), as the *one* sex act that we know must be happening takes place in glowing silhouette.

However, this scene is the two men's initial sexual encounter, which takes place before they love each other and also before Alex discloses his HIV status. It marks several combined unrepresentabilities in the comic. Even sex with someone whom one *will come to love* cannot be explicitly depicted. Visually explicit safer sex is equally illusive. And, in nominally resexualizing the seropositive body, love comes to *replace* sex, as the erotic as a loving, perverse sexual encounter is displaced by the purely affective. We never see Alex and Michel have sex at all after they have declared their love and after Alex has disclosed his HIV status. Michel returns after Alex's disclosure, but what we see thereafter is a kiss and a scene of the two cuddling fully clothed. Seropositive sexuality becomes possible towards the narrative's conclusion only by implication. Removed from the thinkable or representable, it is recouperable only through the reaffirmation of an implicitly monogamous relationship, with its associated normative subject/object divisions and prescribed temporalities. Now, the fear of being cut off from affective relationships is certainly a common post-diagnosis concern. But, here, love exists only through the exclusion of the erotic and even sex. As Haver notes, one of the benefits of the perverse is its ability "to think the contingent encounter of anonymous sexual nomads … to be an act of loving"—one that is certainly unthinkable in a text where casual encounters are only depicted as sites of seroconversion (1996, 142).

Indeed, Crimp notoriously identifies perverse sexuality and promiscuity as queer men's greatest epidemiological tool, arguing that "We were able to invent safe sex because we have always known that sex is not, in an epidemic or not, limited to penetrative sex. Our

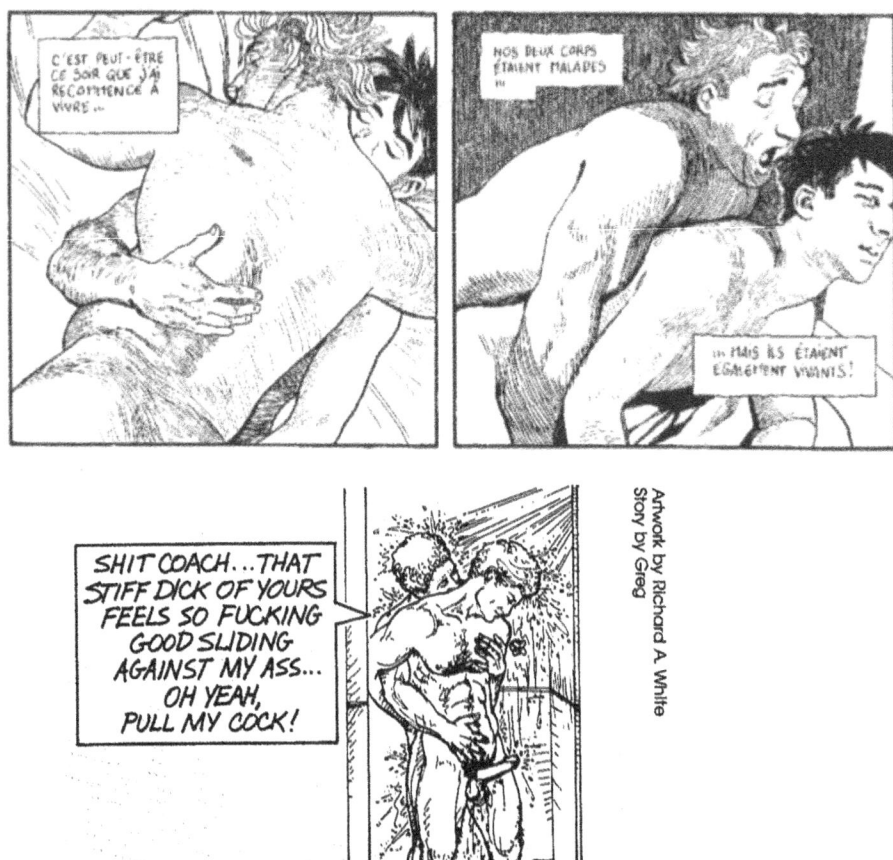

Fig. 6 Above, Alex has sex with Vincent, his first sexual encounter after his (Alex's) diagnosis. Vincent embraces Alex from behind. (Robberecht and Neaud. *Alex*, 26. Courtesy of Ex Aequo, Brussels.); Below, excerpt from *Safer Sex Comix #1*, in which "Coach" embraces his sexual partner from behind. (Story by Greg and artwork by Richard A. White. *Safer Sex Comix #1*. [New York: GMHC Publications, 1986]. Courtesy of Gay Men's Health Crisis, New York)

promiscuity taught us many things, not only about the pleasures of sex, but about the great multiplicity of those pleasures" (1987, 153). Preceding both Patton and, later, Rosengarten, Crimp also argues that sex is, as Patton puts it, "the form of power that makes and saves queer lives" (1996, 155). What has happened, then, between *Safer Sex Comix* and *Alex* when it comes to this life-saving perversity that Patton, Haver, Rosengarten, and Crimp valorize as both culturally crucial and epidemiologically necessary? One of the elements that vanishes is the emphasis on the erotic as, to draw on Haver, a connection between bodies that are neither clean nor proper, where clean and proper bodies are intimately connected to "clean and proper bodies politic" (1996, 12). In the service of the much needed goal of a workable HIV-positive subject position, *Alex* reinstates clean and proper bodily and body political boundaries, prioritizing an affective reclamation of sociality that depends on the renewal of the citizen's normative relational temporality and its associated discursive framing of "sex" as intercourse. Subjects (and objects) solidify in Alex; they do not embrace "erotic congress with the other [as] a matter, *the* matter in its materiality, of flows, of fluids and fluidity, of the radical instability … of flux" (Haver 1996, 12). In *Safer Sex Comix*, however, seemingly minor acts

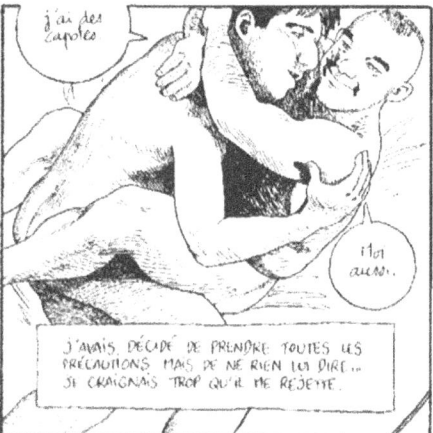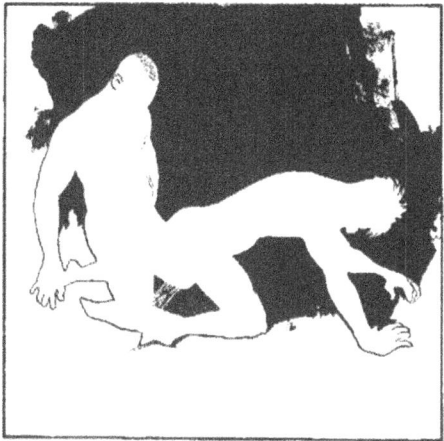

Fig. 7 Alex's first (and only visually depicted) sexual encounter with Michel. Both men appear in glowing silhouette against a dark, patchy spot on an otherwise blank background. (Robberecht and Neaud. *Alex*, 35. Courtesy of Ex Aequo, Brussels)

of stylistic creativity emphasize the ontology of bodies that are always prospectively neither clean not proper, which seek modes of erotic connection that breach self/other boundaries without high-risk fluid exchange.

In *Safer Sex Comix*, there is no distinction between HIV-positive and HIV-negative bodies. Antibody tests for HIV were first approved by the FDA in the US in 1985, and they were not immediately widely used, there or anywhere else; a positive test result had little to offer but anxiety at a time when there were no effective treatments. As such, all characters in GMHC's campaign are prospectively positive or negative and must behave as if they could be either. The sex they explore is equally for the protection and pleasure of both partners, who remain necessarily in a state of subjectivity-complicating indeterminacy. Rather than "the erotic ... conceived ... [as] a simple transaction or negotiation between an unproblematic self and a disgusting but nonetheless unproblematic other, between ontologically primordial entities," the erotic, through the mechanism of breached comics panels, functions as a transaction between bodies that are always already problematic (Haver 1996, 12). With the advent and adoption of HIV-screening, these categories become more distinct (although not entirely, since not every sexually active person gets tested regularly or at all[11]). The return to structures, categories, and orderly bodies and temporalities (e.g. through the affective-temporal framework of monogamous love), is a strategy for reasserting a sense of self for HIV-positive subjects who may experience themselves as untenably disgusting, as can be seen in Alex's dramatic reaction to cutting himself, as well as in the testimonies of the interview participants reproduced at the comic's conclusion—but at the cost of a potential reappropriation of the problematically fluid body, and its fluids, into pleasures beyond the banality of anal.

Indeed, feelings of self-disgust are a major, and important, concern of *Alex*'s. Not only does Alex conceptualize his own potential fluidity through the image of himself as a virus-spewing monster, but also one of the interview participants, Nicolas, states, "J'ai un dégoût de mon corps, de mon sperme, j'ai peur de salir et de contaminer mon compagnon, meme si je sais qu'en nous protégeant, le risqué de transmission est quasi nul"—"I have a disgust with my body, with my sperm; I'm afraid of dirtying and infecting my boyfriend, even if I know that, in protecting ourselves, the risk of transmission is virtually zero" (Robberecht and Neaud 2008,

45). The interviews capture the anxieties of subjectification, permeable bodily boundaries, and self-disgust of their subjects, but they neglect their strategies for negotiating pleasure and desire—and, because the final work does not include the interview questions or the full interviews, it is unclear whether this lack was built in from the outset or the result of later writing and editorial choices. Conversely, *Safer Sex Comix* are able to negotiate effectively visualizing safely and pleasurably breaching subjective boundaries through the metaphorical breaching of panel borders with sexual acts, body parts, and fluids, in part because of the lack of distinction between HIV-positive and negative bodies. While it is neither possible nor desirable to return to the historical moment in which *Safer Sex Comix* were produced, their erotic strategies still have something to contribute to the parallel goals of transmission-reduction and supporting HIV-positive subjectification in the present day.

In particular, the emphasis on come shots as *Safer Sex Comix*'s most frequently depicted perverse pleasure is eroto-philosophically useful, epidemiologically productive, and, in the contemporary context, a potential reinvestment of pleasure in the bodily fluid that fills Nicolas, for example, with so much disgust. Exuberant ejaculation is a mainstay of *Safer Sex Comix*. In Issue 1, the penultimate panel reads: "Bend over and spread em … while my cock shoots this hot wad all over your back!" (Greg and White 1986). Issue 2's penultimate page is a two panel conversation reading, "Oh God … I'm gonna *come* on you!" to which the reply is "here's my *load* too!!", as both partners shoot across the panel borders (Greg and Bodenschatz 1986). Even Issue 3, which depicts phone sex, celebrates ejaculate and ejaculation, as, in the second to last page, each man's come spurts towards the dividing panel line, forming one large splash that belies the division of the comics panel and the spatial separation of the issue's protagonists (Greg and Matt 1986). It is worth noting at this point that, while the writer of each of these issues is the same, the artists are different. Their use of a similar stylistic strategy to approach body fluid, then, indicates the kind of in-community sexual discourse that Patton argues is occluded by dominant discourses of safer sex education, representing a possible site of recuperation of the problematic seropositive body, in all its disorderly fluidity.

The thing that is the most utterly perversely unthinkable—and unthought—in *Alex* is transgressing the boundary that the national discourse asserts between seropositive and assumed to be seronegative bodies, although the text does gesture in this direction through Neaud's failure to draw a dividing line between Alex's and Michel's bodies in their one explicitly, if allusively, depicted sexual encounter (Fig. 7). Patton writes that "most public health officials were convinced that bonding (by serostatus) and not bondage was the best means of halting the transmission of HIV" (1996, 117). And, indeed, there is not a single depiction, in *Alex*, of someone who is seronegative *knowingly* having sex with someone who is seropositive. Drawing the riotous explicit-ness of the indeterminate bodies and fluids from *Safer Sex Comix* into works that address the post-ARV landscape could well aid in both envisioning seropositive sexuality and desire/desirability and responding to more contemporary epidemiological concerns. In contending with the reemergence of unprotected anal intercourse among MSM in recent years, David Halperin proposes abjection as a critical lens in *What Do Gay Men Want?* For him, abjection, while it can potentially lead to risky behavior, does not necessarily have to. As Halperin writes, "Modern postindustrial societies produce social conditions that seem to foster in their citizens yearning for escape, exemption, … self-loss, transcendence. Abjection offers one such opportunity; the voluntary pursuit of risk offers another; pleasure ... holds out a third. It is because risky sex manages to conjoin ... all three of those modes ... that it remains both so seductive and so unmanageable" (2007, 96). The come shot is a form of indigenous perversity that prospectively falls under the category of sexual act or dynamic that Halperin argues could be reclaimed under the auspices of the desirable abject thus defined. While it does not necessarily hold a privileged position, and, indeed, more attentive conversation with MSM about their preferred, non-penetrative erotic practices would undoubtedly reveal other possibilities that perform similar erotic functions, the ubiquity of ejaculating on men's bodies in *Safer Sex Comix* warrants attention. Halperin uses as an example of the sexual abject Jean Genet's description, in *The Thief's Journal*, of the tube of vaseline that his arresting police officers have retrieved from his pocket and mocked; it represents "his filthiness, ... his subordination, his vulnerability, his anal receptivity ..." (Halperin 2007, 81). Ejaculate, in traversing the space between bodies and landing on the body of another, performs a similar function, one that is able to accommodate seropositive bodies and fluids as desirable and erotic without high risk of transmission.

In her canonical *Hard Core*, Linda Williams represents the money shot in heterosexual pornography as striving to visually capture both male and female sexual pleasure (1989, see 180 etc.), but the come shot in *Safer Sex Comix* is neither purely allusive nor purely safer sex strategy but a depiction of an extant sexual practice that pre-dates the AIDS crisis. While abjection, and its erotic potential, is certainly not limited to sadomasochistic practice, *Safer Sex Comix #5* is particularly illuminating here. The dominant sexual partner, whose leather-clad legs and enormous penis already cannot be contained by the panel frame, is desirable in part for his ability to dramatically come *on* not merely *in*, as his sexual partner pleads, "Please, sir, would you shoot your man-cum on my chest?" and is rewarded with a spurt that breaks the border of the following panel (Fig. 1). Here, semen, the source of Nicolas' self-disgust, the risky bodily fluid, is reappropriated as erotic object, existing at the conjunction of abjection, risk, and pleasure as it traverses the distance between bodies, between problematic subjects. Sex that is literally dirty defies the notion of clean and proper bodies and bodies politic. Reclaiming, in Halperin's term, the filthiness of sex, bodies, and sexual subjects through acts that are not epidemiologically risky can help not only to reassert the in- discreet and discrete pleasure of the erotic but also potentially the desirousness and desire of seropositive bodies themselves.

While, in *Alex*, not only does the plenitude of perverse acts that breach the panels of *Safer Sex Comix* disappear into the sex that is just one, but the thing that proves the most unthinkably perverse is to desire a seropositive body, pressing against the thinkable edge of sex's and sexuality's dirtiness has prospective benefits that span the theoretical, the cultural, the philosophical, and the pragmatic. Sex (or knowing sex), perversely erotic or not, with a seropositive partner when one is not "bonding by serostatus" becomes literally unrepresentable in *Alex* in a way that is not necessarily unassailable and whose alteration may well benefit efforts, admirably evident in this project, to address feelings of self-disgust and subjective difficulties post-diagnosis. It is, indeed, the edge of the erotically thinkable, an edge that that could well be approached, and would be well to approach, through more careful considerations of in-community strategies of boundary-breaching, erotic perversion, and sexual variety such as those expressed in the pages of *Safer Sex Comix*.

Acknowledgements This paper has benefited immensely from the support and thoughtful comments and suggestions of the special issue editors, Rebecca Garden and William Spurlin, and the external reviewer.

Endnotes

[1] We might characterize it as a graphic novella: about forty pages plus back matter.

[2] Rosengarten makes this point in "The Challenge of HIV for Feminist Theory" (2004, 213). Along with Eric Mykhalovskiy, she also associates this historical moment with "enhanc [ing] the vulnerability of HIV to [the] closure of thought and inquiry" she identifies in a turn away from discursive and cultural scholarship on HIV, effectively linking the decline in theoretical fecundity after 1996 to its role as a biomedical pivot point (Mykhalovskiy and Rosengarten 2009, 189).

[3] See, particularly, *Law's Desire* and *Governing Sexuality*.

[4] My thanks to my reviewer for pointing out that the emphasis on anal sex in harm reduction material can inspire some people to avoid it. This is certainly true, though it seems to be a minority response. As Dowsett has observed (2009, 231), sexual behavior surveys indicate an increase in the prevalence of anal sex among MSM over the last quarter century, indicating that those scared away by its centrality to safer sex campaigns are less numerous than those who practice it. Dowsett's focus is Australia, but the material he draws from suggests a broader Western trend.

[5] Mainstream/sub-cultural categorization is necessarily complicated. Kramer was a founding member of both GMHC and the AIDS activist group ACT-UP. However, he was ejected from GMHC for his views before *Safer Sex Comix* were published, and *The Normal Heart*, his play about AIDS, which was very critical of MSM sexual cultures, achieved wide-scale praise from the (straight) mainstream.

[6] Most criticisms of PrEP present the greatly diminished risk of seroconversion offered by prophylactic anti-HIV medication as prospectively increasing "promiscuity," echoing conservative US objections to, for example, vaccinating girls against HPV lest it "encourage pre-marital sex."

[7] The story in this issue (and a number of others) is credited to a writer who goes only by "Greg," with no last name provided. Some of the artists are also credited by first name only. *Safer Sex Comix* are not paginated.

[8] All translations mine.

[9] Alex interacts with a number of other positive characters who tell him their stories.

[10] While I do not have space to explore the issue of risk *reduction* rather than risk *avoidance* in this article, *Alex* is consistently opposed to common risk reduction strategies. The comic emphasizes the risks of super- and co-infection, discouraging serosorting. A common risk reduction strategy for MSM who practice unprotected penetrative sex is strategic positioning; since the receptive partner is statistically at greater risk of infection, partners determine sexual role based on HIV status. Alex's infection, as the penetrating partner, implicitly dismisses this strategy. The back matter of the comic emphasizes the risks of unprotected oral sex and penetrative sex with a partner whose viral load is undetectable. While Alex's viral load eventually becomes undetectable, its effect on his risk of transmission is never discussed in the storyspace.

[11] As Rosengarten argues, the introduction of HIV viral load testing, with a possible result of "undetectable," complicates such distinctions even further, as it is then possible to be HIV-positive while having no detectable virus in the peripheral bloodstream (2004, 213).

References

Crimp, Douglas. 1987. "How to have Promiscuity in an Epidemic." *October* 43: 237-271. http://jstor.org/stable/3397576.

Dowsett, Gary W. 2009. "Dangerous Desires and Post-queer HIV Prevention: Rethinking Community, Incitement and Intervention." *Social Theory & Health* 7 (3): 218-240.

Greg and Alexander. 1986. *Safer Sex Comix #5: Leatherman*. New York: GMHC Publications.

Greg and Bill Bodenschatz. 1986. *Safer Sex Comix #2*. New York: GMHC Publications.

Greg and Matt. 1986. *Safer Sex Comix #3*. New York: GMHC Publications.

Greg and Richard A. White. 1986. *Safer Sex Comix #1*. New York: GMHC Publications.

Halperin, David. 2007. *What Do Gay Men Want?: An Essay on Sex, Risk, and Subjectivity*. Ann Arbor: University of Michigan Press.

 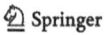

Haver, William. 1996. *The Body of This Death: Historicity and Sociality in the Time of AIDS*. Stanford: Stanford University Press.

Mykhalovskiy, Eric and Marsha Rosengarten. 2009. "HIV/AIDS in its Third Decade: Renewed Critique in Social and Cultural Analysis – An Introduction." *Social Theory & Health* 7 (3): 187-195.

Patton, Cindy. 1996. *Fatal Advice: How Safe-Sex Education Went Wrong*. Durham and London: Duke University Press.

Robbrecht, Thierry and Fabrice Neaud. 2008. *Alex et la vie d'après*. Brussels: Ex Aequo. http://www.exaequo.be/pdf/268-EXA-bd-alex-LD.pdf.

Rosengarten, Marsha. 2004. "The Challenge of HIV for Feminist Theory." *Feminist Theory* 5 (2). https://doi.org/10.1177/1464700104045409.

———. 2009. *HIV Interventions: Biomedicine and the Traffic Between Information and Flesh*. Seattle: University of Washington Press.

Stychin, Carl F. 1995. *Law's Desire: Sexuality and the Limits of Justice*. London/New York: Routledge.

———. 2003. *Governing Sexuality: The Changing Politics of Citizenship and Law Reform*. Oxford: Hart Publishing.

Williams, Linda. 1989. *Hard Core: Power, Pleasure, and the "Frenzy of the Visible."* Berkeley and Los Angeles: University of California Press.

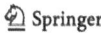

J Med Humanit (2019) 40:53–68
https://doi.org/10.1007/s10912-018-9531-3

Fanon and the New Paraphilias: Towards a Trans of Color Critique of the DSM-V

Stephanie Hsu[1]

Published online: 4 August 2018
© Springer Science+Business Media, LLC, part of Springer Nature 2018

Abstract This essay places psychiatrist and philosopher Frantz Fanon's anti-colonial, anti-racist message from *Peau Noire, Masques Blancs/Black Skin, White Masks* (1952; 1967; 2008) in conversation with the new diagnoses of "Gender Dysphoria" and "Transvestic Disorder" in the fifth edition of the *Diagnostic and Statistical Manual of Mental Disorders* (DSM-V). Specifically, the essay discusses sexologist Ray Blanchard's controversial theory of autogynephilia alongside Fanon's ambivalent rendering of transgender desire and interracial trans phenomenology in a crucial but frequently overlooked passage in *Black Skin*. Fanon's anti-colonial critique of psychiatry allows us to reconsider how Blanchard's theories on paraphilia engage with the foundational psychoanalytic concepts of identification and desire, as identified by the Freudian and Lacanian models and explored in the writings of Judith Butler, Catherine Millot, Charles Shepherdson, and others. By offering a fresh interpretation of the French text, this essay argues that a "trans of color critique" can benefit from *Black Skin*'s unexpected insight into trans desire: Fanon's "man of color," who simultaneously undergoes a gender transition and a racial transformation, represents the literal embodiment of his critique of colonial racism. Given the role of the new paraphilias in the DSM-V, this essay concludes that a trans of color critique is well positioned to reinforce the anti-colonial message Fanon addressed to the psychiatric and psychoanalytical fields, which have tended to diagnose psychic injury while ignoring its causation, and which continue to neglect the fact that medical access is just as important as material support and security for minority subjects, in particular.

Keywords Race · Transgender · Colonialism · Paraphilia · Autogynephilia

The only passage in anti-colonial theorist Frantz Fanon's *Peau Noire, Masques Blancs/Black Skin, White Masks* explicitly to mention a transgender performance of identity appears as a footnote to the book's sixth chapter, "The Negro and Psychopathology" (1952; 1967; 2008). In what has come to be known among postcolonial scholars simply as "footnote 44," Fanon

✉ Stephanie Hsu
  shsu@pace.edu

[1] Pace University, 41 Park Row, 15th Floor, New York, NY 10038, USA

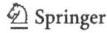

reiterates his famous claim that because the colonized and displaced peoples of the Caribbean have resisted the psychic imprint of the European Oedipus complex, there is no overt practice of homosexuality in Martinique. Yet he also mentions here the well-known existence of Martinican "'men dressed as women' or 'godmothers'" who are not homosexual but "lead normal sex lives" and who, though they cross-dress, seem not to exhibit those psychopathological symptoms of racist injury which interested Fanon as a psychiatrist practicing in French colonial hospitals (1967, 180).

In fact, Fanon reserves his concern for subjects like the speaker in chapter three, "The Man of Color and the White Woman," who narrates these lines:

> I wish to be acknowledged not as *black* but as *white*.
> Now [...] who but a white woman can do this for me? By loving me she proves that I am worthy of white love. I am loved like a white man.
> I am a white man.
> Her love takes me onto the noble road that leads to total realization...
> I marry white culture, white beauty, white whiteness.
> When my restless hands caress those white breasts, they grasp white civilization and dignity and make them mine.[1] (1967, 63)

This phenomenological account of interracial desire testifies to Fanon's belief that colonial racism induces a form of psychosis—that is, a disturbance in the colonized subject's perception of reality (especially with regard to gender identity) to which our current diagnostic categories of dysphoria and dysmorphia roughly correspond.[2] For Fanon, the psychic injury of colonization carries a disembodying force that divides the speaker from his skin even as it reduces his lover to the shape of "those white breasts." In this description of interracial love and eroticism, however, we can also detect an *implicit* reference to trans identity and a desire for trans embodiment which is more clearly conveyed by the original French, as I will show.[3] Although existing English translations of *Black Skin* do not render this interpretation, Fanon's narrator is not only fantasizing in this passage about a somatic transition from black to white but also from male to female. Although footnote 44 makes it clear that Fanon did not regard cross-dressing or other forms of gender variant self-presentation to be inherently problematic, the relationship he depicts between the man of color and the white woman appears to mobilize the psychoanalytical paradigms of desire and identification in ways that do indeed produce what he considered to be psychopathology.

This essay places *Black Skin*'s anti-colonial, anti-racist message in conversation with emergent diagnostic approaches to trans identity and transvestism in the fifth edition of the *Diagnostic and Statistical Manual of Mental Disorders* (DSM-V), released by the American Psychiatric Association in May 2013. Specifically, I discuss sexologist Ray Blanchard's controversial theory of autogynephilia, which—to the consternation of trans activists, including the World Professional Association for Transgender Health—has been included in the diagnostic criteria for "Transvestic Disorder" and classified as a "Paraphilia" or a "Sexual Dysfunction" in the DSM-V. Autogynephilia, defined by Blanchard as "the love of oneself as a woman," and its symmetrical counterpart, autoandrophilia, forward a dramatically new version of erotically-motivated gender transition that, to my view, bears an uncanny resemblance to Fanon's phenomenology of interracial desire (2005, 439). Because Fanon regarded his patients' symptoms as real and embodied responses to social oppression, however, the similarity between his conception of trans desire and that of the Sexual and Gender Identity Disorders

Work Group, the DSM-V revision committee appointed by the American Psychiatric Association, offers an opportunity to bring anti-racist and anti-colonial perspectives to bear upon the new diagnoses of paraphilia. In spite of his own lack of familiarity with trans issues, Fanon's insights allow us to critique the colonizing force of the DSM-V in its tendency to isolate the notion of mental disorder from its full range of cultural, socio-economic, and political contexts—not to mention its daring to expand medical knowledge at the risk of contributing to the pathologization of trans experience, in particular.

Certainly, such a critique is not in itself unprecedented. As recently as 2010, a study concluded that the American Psychiatric Association's influence over global health policy has promoted worldwide a medicalized model of trans identity which makes gender variant populations' access to health care dependent on the DSM-IV's diagnosis of "Gender Identity Disorder" (GID) (Vance, Jr. et al.). In other words, individuals may have to obtain a GID diagnosis not only to receive gender transition-related treatment but also to access basic medical care that is appropriate for their bodies. Conducted by a team of researchers that included Kenneth J. Zucker, the chair of the DSM-V's Sexual and Gender Identity Disorders Work Group, this international survey of community-based, transgender support organizations revealed a broad consensus around the stigmatizing nature of GID and provided a clear demonstration of the American Psychiatric Association's neocolonial reach: over half of the community organizations responding to the survey believed that GID should be removed from the DSM altogether, and those who opposed or were uncertain as to the removal of GID also reported that the diagnosis is in fact required by legal or medical authorities in those countries (Vance, Jr. et al 2010).[4]

Having first entered the DSM-III in 1980 in connection to the diagnosis of "Transsexualism" before replacing the latter in all future editions, GID was therefore an early target for revision by Zucker's DSM-V Work Group, which quickly determined that GID would be replaced by the less-stigmatizing term "Gender Dysphoria" in the upcoming fifth edition (American Psychiatric Association 2012). This shift from the notion of an identity-based disorder to an impairment-based concept such as dysphoria has been hailed as a victory for the trans rights movement by the news media and in lesbian, gay, bisexual, transgender, and queer (LGBTQ) community circles. However, as trans activist Julia Serano (2012) and others have protested, Zucker's Work Group also decided to include Blanchard's novel concepts of autogynephilia and autoandrophilia under the banner of Transvestic Disorder, a diagnosis that links cross-dressing to erotic ideation and sexual arousal in ways which do not add to our understanding of gender variance so much as expand our definition of sexual dysfunction or deviance (American Psychiatric Association 2012). And in what would appear to be a major conflict of interest—or what Fanon would surely have us regard as a nepotistic distribution of colonial power—appointed to serve on this very same DSM-V Work Group was Blanchard himself.

Autogynephilia in the new "transvestic disorder" diagnosis

In 1989, Blanchard defined autogynephilia as "the love of oneself as a woman" and proposed this concept as the key to identifying an "erotic orientation" in cross-dressing individuals. Blanchard was a clinical sexologist at an institution treating sex offenders in Toronto when he attained this "perceptual shift [...] in the way I saw, heard, and understood statements that patients had been making to clinicians for decades," he states (2005, 439). What he perceived was a difference between a subject who admits "that he is sexually excited by wearing a brassiere" and one who admits "that he is sexually excited by the idea of having breasts" (2005, 445). The former statement comports with the long-standing diagnostic criteria for "Transvestic Fetishism," which the DSM defined in the 1980s as a disorder exclusively affecting heterosexual males, and it also correlates with the cross-dressing culture popularized by heterosexual-identified white men in the U.S. starting in the 1960s (Stryker 2008). Finding this medicalized approach to cross-dressing lacking in its focus on literal clothing rather than erotic ideation, e.g., "the idea of having breasts," Blanchard reflects, "I therefore reluctantly concluded that I had no alternative but to invent a new word" (2005, 444).

With established researcher Kurt Freund, Blanchard began publicizing the notion of autogynephilia in connection with another of his original notions: "developmental errors of erotic target location" (1993). Most evident in heterosexual men, erotic target localization error is

a theory [which] predicts that, for every class of sexual object, there will be small subgroups of men who develop fetishes for clothing associated with the desired object, who develop the erotic fantasy of being the desired object, and who develop the sustained wish to transform their own bodies into facsimiles of the desired object. (Freund and Blanchard 1993, 562)

Blanchard's theory of erotic motivation suggests a continuum of non-normative self-fashioning practices that resembles the spectrum-based models of gender identity and expression currently in use in LGBTQ grassroots discourse but for one glaring difference: the "desired object" in his theory is always determined by a heterosexual orientation.[5] His insistence on classifying cross-dressers and trans individuals first and foremost as either heterosexual or homosexual with reference to their original gender assignment at birth carries on a sexological tradition which he himself traces to Magnus Hirschfeld's first mention of transvestism in 1910 (Freund and Blanchard 1993). It also conflates gender identity and sexual orientation as categories of social formation which contemporary queer theory, for its part, has tried to keep separate through a critique of compulsory heterosexuality and its attendant gender norms.

In fact, by proposing that gender variance results from overshooting one's actual erotic target—that some trans women, for instance, are men who love women too much—autogynephilia subverts the real diversity of lived gender experience and subordinates it to the logic of compulsory heterosexuality. This logic allows Blanchard to attribute a predictive force to his particular understanding of eroticism, which takes a deterministic view of the progression from cross-dressing to transsexualism: "As a practical matter, the autogynephilic type seems to have a higher risk of developing gender dysphoria," he counsels researchers and clinicians (2010, 368). As other sexologists took up his work, autoandrophilia or "the love of oneself as a man" was peremptorily coined to serve as autogynephilia's exact counterpart in subjects assigned female at birth, but virtually no studies into autoandrophilia have been completed. On the basis of Blanchard's limited findings, the Sexual and Gender Identity Disorders Work Group nonetheless proposed two major revisions to the DSM-IV's classification of Transvestic Fetishism in order to establish the new diagnosis of Transvestic Disorder: first, they removed the criterion that limited the diagnosis to heterosexual males; and secondly, they required patients to specify whether they are sexually aroused by fabrics, materials, or garments ("With Fetishism"), or by the thought of image of self as female/male ("With Autogynephilia"/"With Autoandrophilia") (American Psychiatric Association 2012).

Although Blanchard has suggested that autogynephilia and autoandrophilia belong on a continuum with gender dysphoria, Transvestic Disorder in the DSM-V in fact forwards an alternate etiology or medical model of trans identity which draws upon an older logic of paraphilia. Pertaining to sexual arousal generated by objects or situations that are deemed non-normative, paraphilia has been synonymous with sexual deviation since the initial 1952 edition of the DSM and included cross-dressing among its earliest examples. Autogynephilia and autoandrophilia are treated as new paraphilias because they regard the desire for trans embodiment as co-extensive with sexual arousal at the idea of *being* the desired object: in the context of practicing a "love of oneself as a woman," the object of desire is none other than femininity itself. For proponents of Blanchard's theories, paraphilic desire seems to offer a refreshing alternative to the distressing "wrong body narrative" which dominates our under-standing of dysphoria (Stone 1987), and they have enthusiastically taken to promoting autogynephilia as the hidden or authoritative truth of trans women's experience.

Trans-identified sexologist Anne Lawrence (1999), for instance, claims that "autogynephilic eroticism is not just an incidental finding, but is rather the central motivation for the transsexual journey." Characterizing gender dysphoria as an "outmoded idea" which is perpetuated by the medical establishment, she declares, "If we make it clear that we regard paraphilic arousal to feminization as consistent with genuine transsexualism, then our clients will probably tell us the truth" rather than "simply tell[ing] us precisely what we want to hear—just as they have done for decades" (Lawrence 1999).[6] Intersex researcher Alice Dreger, who has defended not only Blanchard's ideas but also the controversial work of his colleague, J. Michael Bailey, similarly argues: "Although the [wrong body] narrative may function socially and clinically like a sort of get-out-of-male-free card, this pushing of sex into the closet where transsexuality is concerned at some level robs transwomen of their erotic possibilities and realities" (2008, 416). Both Lawrence and Dreger suggest that by expanding the notion of "genuine transsexualism" beyond the criteria for GID or Gender Dysphoria, we might reverse the power dynamic between patients and medical professionals and make room instead for the truth about trans eroticism. However, the very idea that there could be a genuine or singular trans experience appears to have sparked something of a rivalry between the new paraphilias and the established version of dysphoria in the DSM-V, and the evolving stakes of this contest may not come down to which diagnosis is the more truthful but rather which will prove to be the least stigmatizing to trans people.

For activists like Julia Serano, Transvestic Disorder in the DSM-V does not incarnate a closet from which expressions of trans eroticism might emerge but functions instead as a backdoor diagnosis that continues to validate the surveillance and the unnecessary pathologization of gender variant individuals. Although Serano has been speaking and writing on the topic of "why feminists should be concerned with the impending revision of the DSM" since 2009, she notes her puzzlement at the apparent lack of community reaction to Transvestic Disorder, especially since the concept of autogynephilia drew public fire when it was introduced nearly fifteen years ago in J. Michael Bailey's *The Man Who Would Be Queen* (2003), a work of popular science that has been compared to Janice Raymond's *The Transsexual Empire* (1979) in its delegitimizing of trans identity (Serano 2012). In applying Blanchard's theories to his own interviews with trans women, Bailey indeed shows how the concept of autogynephilia can produce heterosexist assumptions about trans desire as well as reproduce heterosexist valuations of femininity. He writes, for instance, "There is no way to say this as sensitively as I would prefer, so I will just go ahead. Most homosexual transsexuals are much better looking than most autogynephilic transsexuals" (qtd. in Dreger 2008, 382).[7] This sexist or transmisogynistic observation suggests that a theory of erotic motivation could actually reinforce the power imbalance between clinicians or researchers and trans patients whose motives for gender transition would therefore be directly subject to erotic sensibilities not their own. Blanchard's "autogynephilic type"—the person who is sexually aroused from the idea of having breasts, in his original formulation—may be a documented phenomenon, but treating paraphilic desire as a preferred alternative to the wrong body narrative seems likely to result in another round of patients telling doctors what they want to hear, only with far more personal (and eroticized) implications.[8]

Why then have critiques of Transvestic Disorder gained little traction in either LGBTQ activist or queer academic discourse? Serano readily admits, "Personally, I stopped writing about it because I felt like the community was simply not concerned" (2012). Rather than a simple lack of concern, I want to suggest that Transvestic Disorder in the DSM-V has elicited confusion due to the radical shift it represents in the medicalization of trans identity—namely, the superseding of the dysphoria model and the reintroduction of a contested discourse about sexual desire, eroticism, and even love. As Lawrence argues, "historically, the paraphilias often have been regarded as exclusively erotic phenomena, and those who experience them have been assumed not to be fully capable of love" (2007, 512). Because the resulting "social bias against paraphilic sexuality" has also fueled intolerance of cross-dressing practices and contributed to the ideology of transphobia, she declares that autogynephilia must be properly recognized as an "'amatory propensity,'" a "special type of sexual orientation," and a "variant form of heterosexuality" in order to restore respectability to this class of paraphilic individual (2007, 511). Brooking no distinction between eroticism and love, Lawrence explains that "whatever their preferred targets, these men [...] erroneously locate those erotic targets wholly or partially *inside* themselves, in contrast to the usual pattern of locating erotic targets exclusively outside oneself" (2007, 510). Blanchard's hypothetical subset of trans people are fully capable of love, she concludes—they just seem to have trouble telling their own bodies apart from those of their beloveds.

Fanonian paraphilia

In light of Blanchard's theories, Fanon's brief exploration of trans desire seems all the more striking or prescient, and given how silent Blanchard and his supporters have been about the impact of race or ethnicity on their research into erotically-motivated gender transition, the need to recur to Fanon's insight is all the more urgent. In the passage from "The Man of Color and the White Woman" with which I began, Fanon throws his voice like a ventriloquist in order to propose that because he is loved like a white man, he can be elliptically identified as a white man. It is not difficult to imagine that Fanon was thinking of his own wife—Marie-Josèphe "Josie" Dublé, a white French journalist who married him in 1952, just as *Black Skin* was being published—when he proclaims at an earlier moment in the book, "Today, I believe in the possibility of love; that is why I endeavor to trace its imperfections, its perversions" (1967, 42). Yet his loving perversions are precisely what Fanon's translators have failed to capture fully. Here again is how Charles Lam Markmann first interpreted this portion of the text in the 1967 Grove Press edition, followed by Fanon's original lines.

> Her love takes me onto the noble road that leads to total realization...
> I marry white culture, white beauty, white whiteness.
> When my restless hands caress those white breasts, they grasp white civilization and dignity and make them mine. (63)

Son amour m'ouvre l'illustre couloir qui mène à la prégnance totale…
J'épouse la culture blanche, la beauté blanche, la blancheur blanche.
Dans ces seins blancs que mes mains ubiquitaires caressent, c'est la
civilisation et la dignité blanches que je fais miennes. (1952, 51)

These lines are interpreted in a nearly identical manner by Richard Philcox in his translation for the 2008 reissue of *Black Skin*:

Her love opens the illustrious path that leads to total fulfillment…
I espouse white culture, white beauty, white whiteness.
Between these white breasts that my wandering hands fondle, white civilization and worthiness become mine. (45)

While both English translations offer the hypostasized figure of "white whiteness" as an overt expression of the speaker's interracial desire, the original text displays an ambiguity which gives rise in at least two places to what I perceive as the speaker's ambivalent desire for trans embodiment. The final sentence of this passage, for instance, contains a sylleptic logic that Markmann and Philcox each gloss differently based on their interpretation of the French preposition *dans*, which can indicate either a physical or a figurative location. As Markmann's translation demonstrates more clearly, the syntactic proximity between "white breasts" and "white civilization or dignity" implies that the actions of caressing and grasping equally confer possession: his speaker seems be saying that white dignity, white civilization, and white breasts *are all made mine*. Philcox's translation strains sense by locating white privilege in a tangible place, i.e., literally between a white woman's breasts, while Markmann's temporal clause ("When my restless hands") points to the continuous availability of the female body to affirm the speaker's desired racial identification and to ground his iterative claim to heterosexuality. Either way, the English versions avoid dealing with the ubiquitous agency of Fanon's hands ("*mes mains ubiquitaires*"), which they characterize instead as "restless" or "wandering." By de-emphasizing the role that the speaker plays in actively conjuring the female form which he perceives, Markmann and Philcox depict the female body as passive and inert, and yet her love ("*Son amour*") is described as the motivating force that euphemistically leads him down the "noble road to total realization" or the "illustrious path that leads to total fulfillment."

In fact, these initial lines suggest that our speaker imagines himself to be more than just a man of color with (white) breasts. Both English translations treat "*la prégnance totale*" in the manner that Maurice Merleau-Ponty, Fanon's erstwhile teacher, used the gestalt concept of pregnance to describe a sensory world immanent in its meaning. This world is perceptually available to a consciousness which is implicitly gendered as masculine, and in Fanon's adaptation of this phenomenological framework, whiteness would also appear to be a quality of this consciousness, since the colonial subject's access to meaningful forms of social capital and life experience is only possible upon his assimilation to French culture. If we take *prégnance* literally, however, then Fanon's man of color is becoming fertile, productive, and impregnated through the white woman's love: it is opening a birth canal (since *couloir* often denotes enclosed passages or bounded corridors) in his body as he transitions from black to white and from male, it seems, to female. Although Markmann and Philcox cannot avoid reproducing in part the sylleptic logic that endows Fanon's speaker with breasts in the paradigmatic autogynephilic fantasy, both translators ignore this double entendre about pregnancy which serves to drive home Fanon's description of his black narrator's total unmanning.

For Fanon, this blurring of bodily attributes is symbolic or symptomatic of an interracial desire that reveals how the self-Other relation has been conditioned by the power and privations of the colonial relation. Colonization also carries the force of compulsory hetero-sexual desire in his account, which emphasizes the violence underlying masculine possession and feminine submission and implies that interracial relationships might be as irresistible as they are potentially injurious. Against Lawrence's defense of paraphilic sexuality as a form of romantic love, this fleeting moment of trans embodiment in *Black Skin* therefore depicts the perversion of the black man's love for the white woman. The boundary between their bodies dissolves as the black man loses his racial identity, and "white whiteness" becomes the object of desire which diverts, derails, and ultimately refracts his sexual attraction to the female body back upon himself. In demonstrating the resemblance between Fanon's speaker and Blanchard's autogynephilic type, however, my interpretation of this passage yields an additional, unexpected insight: the man of color who simultaneously undergoes a gender transition and a racial transformation emerges as the literal embodiment of Fanon's critique of colonial racism.

Fanon never resumes this abortive exploration of interracial trans phenomenology in *Black Skin* and exhorts his reader instead to "remember that our purpose is to make possible a healthy encounter between black and white" (1967, 80). In this way, Fanon's man of color voices the unspoken role of race and racism in the current debate over the new paraphilias: what appears unhealthy, so to speak, about the concept of autogynephilia lies not in the wish for trans embodiment itself; rather, how Blanchard and his supporters theorize the relationship between the self and the desired other might be described as unhealthy because they have removed this relation from the social and material contexts in which Fanon locates the source of all psychopathology. In specific terms, Blanchard and his supporters ignore the psycho-analytic approaches to social and material loss that form the foundation of Fanon's anti-colonial and anti-racist thought. Lawrence has described paraphilic sexuality as a confusion between inside and outside, while Blanchard has made reference to "the fusion of the longing to *have* a woman and the longing to *be* a woman—the confounding of desire and envy—which is often apparent in clinical interviews with autogynephiles" (2005, 440). Yet Blanchard himself has confounded here the formula of "having" versus "being" which psychoanalytic theory has consistently posited as the interaction between desire and identification, not desire and envy. By replacing the psychoanalytic concept of identification with the commonplace notion of envy, Blanchard invites a Fanonian critique of his research into trans desire, love, and loss and inadvertently opens the door to another mode of cultural criticism known as "trans of color critique."[9]

Racial envy and trans desire in psychoanalytic theory

"'Autogynephilia' is a sex-fueled mental illness made up by Ray Blanchard," trans activist Andrea James has declared (2004), but Blanchard's own best defense has been that "the study of autogynephilia is, more than anything else, the study of what people *say* about their experiences" (2005, 439). Based on these first-hand accounts, he is able to claim that "the idea of having women's breasts appears to arise quite often in autogynephilic fantasy" (440). The breast, however, also has pride of place in psychoanalytic accounts of ego development and identity formation, as illustrated here in Sigmund Freud's posthumously-published working notes.

> "Having" and "being" in children. [...] Children like expressing an object-relation by an identification: "I am the object." "Having" is the later of the two; after loss of the object it relapses into "being." Example: the breast. "The breast is part of me, I am the breast." Only later: "I have it"—that is, "I am not it." (1964, 47)

Freud refers to the breast as the first object of desire as well as the first lost object, the absence of which makes future forms of identification possible for the child. The loss of the breast is concurrent with the emergence of the child's ego because upon separation from the mother, the breast comes to represent all that the child is not. The ego learns to cope with the subsequent loss of desired objects by changing itself to preserve and resemble what it has loved through processes that Freud calls mourning and melancholia (an incomplete form of mourning). Freud's logic of identification—that we cannot *be* something and *have* that thing at the very same time—therefore poses a fundamental challenge to Blanchard's assertion that autogynephilic men are compelled to identify as trans women because they have erroneously located an external object of desire (say, the breast) inside of themselves or within the boundaries of the bodily ego. More specifically, being precedes having in Freud's scenario, meaning that an initial fantasy to *be* someone ("'I am the object'") is lost and mourned so that one can eventually *have* an identity that reflects this earlier desirous attachment ("'I have it'— that is, 'I am not it'"). Blanchard's description of autogynephiles, however, appears to model the inverse: the desire to *have* a woman as a sexual partner comes before the desire to *be* her in a physical or embodied sense.

The stakes of deploying the concept of envy in an analysis of trans desire become clearer once we compare this possessive and sexually-charged description of autogynephilic envy to Freud's notion of melancholia. While mourning corresponds to a successfully concluded process of ego formation, melancholia represents an incomplete or ongoing state of identification with a desired other. In the case of a melancholic attachment, the subject does not consciously know what has been lost and what should be mourned, and because she resists the realization of loss, any possibility of relating to her desired object also remains foreclosed. Envy, however, presumes that the subject knows exactly what is missing or lacking in herself because both the appearance and the location of the desired object is evidenced by the presence of a rival subject. Blanchard's notion of trans envy entails this simultaneity of possessing the rival woman and communing with her in a state of identity that does not acknowledge loss at all, especially not the loss of what some theorists call the function of sexual difference, as I discuss below. The man of color in *Black Skin* also portrays himself as standing only to gain from his wished-for transformation into the rival white female, but this motivation is furnished by the ideology of racism, which has already determined his blackness to be a personal liability that requires compensation. Implying that envy is synonymous with psychic injury, Fanon suggests that it is the disavowal of loss, the staging of the loss of loss, that inevitably frames his relationship to the white woman's body as an imperial acquisition that can only reproduce the appropriative violence of the colonial encounter.

Despite the argument that a diagnosis of paraphilia could potentially expand medical access to trans and cross-dressing individuals, Blanchard's depiction of trans desire as envious therefore bears weighty ethical implications. In fact, the DSM-IV explicitly distanced itself from any such notion by defining GID as "a strong and persistent cross-gender identification (not merely a desire for any perceived cultural advantages of being the other sex)" (American Psychiatric Association 2000).[10] The portrayal of trans desire as a form of rivalry with cisgender (i.e., non-transgender) women also reprises some of second-wave feminism's most reactionary responses to trans inclusion, including Janice Raymond's accusation that trans women utilize male privilege to appropriate cisgender women's bodies and their political spaces while retaining access to both gendered worlds (1979). As Fanon's work anticipates, the notion of envy or rivalry has also left its mark on critical discourse, particularly in the field of queer studies, about trans women of color.

Take, for instance, the well-known discussions by bell hooks (1992), Judith Butler (1993), and Jay Prosser (1998) about Venus Xtravaganza, one of the documentary subjects of Jennie Livingston's 1991 film on New York City's underground drag ball culture, *Paris is Burning*. A trans youth of color, Venus is a member of the House of Xtravaganza, and her surname announces her belonging in an informal kinship system organized by participation among multiple Houses in runway-style fashion and dance competitions which feature highly creative elements of gender and class-based performance and play. In his influential reading of *Paris*, trans scholar Prosser refers to Venus's "light-skinned Latina transsexual body under construction as heterosexual and female" (1998, 47). In hooks's review of the film, however, Venus is simply a "fair-skinned" figure caught in the community's central conflict over authenticity and racial assimilation: "What viewers witness is not black men longing to impersonate or even to become like 'real' black women, but their obsession with an idealized fetishized vision of femininity that is white" (1992, 154, 148). Venus's race, gender, and sexuality are all treated as points of contention in a debate about the politics of performative identities and the proper parameters for the social recognition of trans women of color in the ball scene and beyond.

In a terrible tragedy, Venus is murdered during the filming of *Paris*, allegedly by one of her dates through an escort service. In the interview sequence which has come to memorialize her, Venus describes herself as "something perfect and little" with blonde hair and green eyes, and she playfully compares her own sexual exchanges with men to those of a suburban housewife who is in quest of a new washer and dryer unit from her husband. In a reading that clearly misses Venus's sardonic commentary on marriage and domesticity here, Butler concludes:

> Now Venus, Venus Xtravaganza, she seeks a certain transubstantiation of gender in order to find an imaginary man who will designate a class and race privilege that promises a permanent shelter from racism, homophobia, and poverty [...] If Venus wants to become a woman, and cannot overcome being a Latina, then Venus is treated by the symbolic in precisely the ways in which women of color are treated [...] In this sense, the "identification" is composed of a denial, an envy, which is the envy of a phantasm of black women, an idealization that produces a denial. (1993, 130-32)

Venus's desire for trans embodiment seems to correspond to a fantasy that "falsely constitutes black [and Latina] women as a site of privilege," Butler continues, and "[h]er death thus testifies to a tragic misreading of the social map of power" (1993, 131). Envy serves as the code word in Butler's analysis for the trans woman of color's state of false consciousness, for an "idealization" of femininity that denies the actual tolls of racism and sexism upon women of color. What Butler herself overlooks, however, is that Venus's identification with this idealized femininity is material and not just phantasmatic, since Venus clearly states that she can pass for white in real life, as she does in the ball scene. In fact, we might expect that Venus *would* be envious of an imagined white woman's "permanent shelter" from oppression when it is homeless queers of color who make up the familial ranks of the House of Xtravaganza. As Sianne Ngai has pointed out, "envy lacks cultural recognition as a valid mode of publicly recognizing or responding to social disparities, even though it remains the *only* agonistic emotion defined as having a perceived inequality as its object" (2005, 128). Venus's envy—like that of Fanon's narrator—might in fact register a political critique of material inequality rather than a merely imagined identification with white femininity though her desire for trans embodiment certainly cannot be separated from her lifelong experience of the latter.

Although racial hierarchy is itself an explicit manifestation of rivalry, envy has proven less productive a concept than melancholic loss for critical race scholars who have claimed Fanon's anti-colonial legacy. For example, in a footnote to her book, *Racial Melancholia*, Anne Cheng credits Fanon with being "the first to gesture toward the reconceptualization of race as melancholic, even though he never talks specifically about melancholia" (2001, 201n24). David L. Eng and Shinhee Han discuss racial melancholia in relation to "assimilation into mainstream culture for people of color [which] still means adopting a set of dominant norms and ideals [...] often foreclosed to them" in the U.S. context where an authentic Asianness and an idealized Americanness can equally function as lost, foreclosed, or impossible objects of desire and identification (2003, 344). However, Eng and Han also observe that there are "losses [which] are grieved because they are not, perhaps, even seen as losses but are seen as social gains," and they offer as an example the loss of parental love objects which furnishes the "foundation of oedipalization" and establishes normative forms gender and sexuality (2003, 362). By rewording this observation slightly, we can recognize that the concept of social gain might also correspond to psychic losses which are *ungrievable* precisely because they do not consciously register as social, cultural, or material loss. For this reason, Butler has claimed that compulsory heterosexuality's foreclosure of same-sex or homogenderal object choice both maintains the borders of normative masculinity and femininity and makes "gender melancholics of us all" (1997, 164).

In the scene of the mutual constitution of race and gender that Fanon's speaker imagines, multiple ungrievable losses are restaged and represented as envious desires. Like Blanchard's autogynephile, Fanon imagines both having *and* being the white woman: this is a seemingly protean state of identity, one unshaped by the ego's defenses against the loss or lack which defines racialized and gendered being. In a social rather than a psychic sense, however, this vision of trans embodiment also represents an incorporation of one's rival according to a formulation of envy that entails wanting *to be* someone in order *to have* what that person has. While Blanchard and his colleagues argue that envy reflects a genuine erotic experience and supports a viable form of paraphilic attachment, Fanon productively associates this same affect with the ideology and message of institutionalized racism: you have *to be* white in order *to have* power, wealth, and security. Herein lie the relative shortcomings of theories about racial and gender melancholia which have nonetheless looked to Fanon's work for support: while melancholia provides a theoretical foundation for normative identities, envy is deemed pathological precisely because it is more political or, in Ngai's wording, "polemical" in its fixation on a specific distribution of social gains rather than a generalized principle of loss—as if minority subjects do not know, as Venus did, exactly what it is that they are being denied (2005, 21).

The contentious status of trans desire across various medico-juridical and cultural discourses therefore reflects a broader, long-standing conflation of the psychoanalytic concept of desire with social or material needs, wants, or demands. For instance, the prohibition formerly associated with GID in the DSM-IV against transitioning one's gender based on "a desire for any perceived cultural advantages of being the other sex" effectively ignores trans people's social and material needs altogether, and it has had the lasting effect of promoting dysphoria as the default condition and the only legitimate motivation for choosing one's gender identity.[11] Fanon, however, posits a causal relationship between psychic disturbances (like dysphoria) and social oppression, or between psychic desires and material losses. This logic of direct causation structured the colonial context in which he practiced, and it has perhaps found a new application in mental health approaches to gender variance today, particularly where trans people of color are concerned. Although Blanchard has contradicted much existing trans scholarship and has failed to engage critical race scholarship at all, his theory of autogynephilia might be turned towards a more productive exploration of the kind of envy that Fanon describes—an envy which can be treated not just as an individualized symptom, but also as a collective index of inequality.

Trans desire in its psychic as well as its social or material guises has consistently posed a unique challenge to traditional schools of psychoanalytic thought, which have tended to associate the attainment of one's desire with modes of psychic suffering—with death or silence, to reference Freud's and Jacques Lacan's models, respectively—rather than with lasting or genuine states of fulfillment. Counterintuitive as it may sound, this perspective on psychopathology tries to account for the intersubjective and mutable grounds of desire itself, which hold a special risk for trans individuals according to the controversial Lacanian analyst, Catherine Millot. Millot's study of transvestism and transsexualism, *Horsexe*, was first published in French in 1983 and was almost universally panned by U.S. trans scholars for its skepticism towards trans desire and its opposition to gender confirming surgeries, in particular (Shepherdson 2000). Since then, scholars such as Gordene Olga MacKenzie have selectively reread *Horsexe* for its salient critique of the medicalization of trans desire. Following Millot, MacKenzie writes, "transsexuals have replaced their desire with the desire of the 'other,' meaning the desires of a bipolar culture achieved through medical science" (1994, 147). Characterizing "the desire of the 'other'" as a rival form of desire, MacKenzie suggests that medical science itself is responsible for generating the motivation to transition and for depicting the surgically-modified body not as an extension of trans desire but as object of envy to be possessed if at all possible. "By subordinating personal 'desire' to cultural 'desire,'" MacKenzie sums up bleakly, "do surgical transsexuals become incapable of experiencing true pleasure [...]?" (1994, 147).

How to tell the difference between one's own desire and the desire of the other would seem to present a fundamental problem for any person, as Shanna T. Carlson conveys when she argues that "'transsexuality' is not in and of itself any more extreme a type of symptom than is 'man' or 'woman'" (2010, 64-65). Yet Charles Shepherdson (2000) has claimed that there are in fact individuals who should not be forwarded as candidates for gender confirming medical procedures—namely, people who resemble Blanchard's autogynephiles. Writing to reinterpret some of Millot's most controversial claims in 1994, roughly ten years after *Horsexe* and five years after Blanchard coined autogynephilia, Shepherdson also invokes the notion of envy or rivalry in his discussion of trans people who identify with an idealized masculine or feminine type and therefore nurture "a fantasy of the 'other sex' as not lacking":

> [T]he subjects who maintain this relation of fantasy to the "other sex" as not lacking, have their subjective consistency precisely on the basis of this relation, this quasi-symbolic link [...] For them, an operation eliminates this point of reference, replacing *a relation to the other* (a symbolic link), however precarious, with *a condition of*

"*being*" that is outside the symbolic, so that surgery, far from liberating them for a future, will on the contrary imprison them once and for all in a position of foreclosure that has been kept at bay only by this fantasy of the other sex. For these subjects, surgery will precipitate a psychotic break. (2000, 109-10)

Reiterating a familiar opposition, Shepherdson compares *having* this "quasi-symbolic link" to an idealized other and *being* "outside the symbolic" altogether after an event like surgery. For trans individuals who do have a fantasy of the "other sex," feelings of envy may constitute a viable if "precarious" relation to sexual difference that nonetheless preserves the possibility of desire's continual movement and circulation. The risk of a "psychotic break," however, might proceed from the challenge of living up to fantasies about an idealized being or accompany the expectation that surgery will have solved all of life's problems. Shepherdson therefore stresses that transitioning one's gender should correspond to changing one's symbolic relationship to sexual difference rather than transcending lack or loss, once and for all. It is only when the rivalry is settled, so to speak, and when desire is no longer possible because its object has been attained that one risks the pathology of *horsexe*, i.e. being "outside sex."

If envy is the affect that characterizes a wish to exist "outside sex," then *Black Skin*'s depiction of a trans desire that is fueled by white envy could be read as an extended meditation on the wish—utopian or dystopian, depending on one's perspective—to exist "outside race" as well. Playing out a fantasy in which the "other race" is not lacking, Fanon's speaker manipulates autogynephilic logic in such a way as to suggest that a person of color cannot *but* become envious over the colonial distribution of racial privilege. Indeed, in the passage from chapter three, it is Fanon's envy and, by extension, his ambivalent desire for trans embodiment that together represent the narrator's precarious link, in Shepherdson's words, to *Black Skin*'s overall vision of social justice. Tim Dean has argued that "articulating psychoanalysis with politics depends upon differentiating between losses and deficits that represent unequal distribution of resources [...] and losses and deficits that are constitutive" of subjectivity as such (2000, 205). By productively confounding these losses, Fanon invites us to wonder which subjects might actually be in a position to tell the difference between the two. Inspired by Fanon, a mode of cultural criticism centering on the experiences of trans people of color might therefore not concern itself with differentiating between psychic injury and social or material inequality at all—indeed, a trans of color critique might even regard the conflation of these terms as productive of an holistic approach to mental health, since redressing the unequal distribution of resources would be tantamount to treating the sources of so-called psychopathology.

Conclusion: towards a trans of color critique of the DSM-V

The question of whether envy is a problematic affect to mobilize in the service of gaining greater access to medical care for trans individuals remains an urgent one, especially since paraphilic eroticism is positioned in the DSM-V to become yet another compulsory narrative for gender variant individuals seeking this access. Indeed, this question points to the unstable ground of advocacy and activism in a so-called post-identity age: are there inherent social, political, or mental wellness-related risks entailed in attempting to deny, transcend, or ignore the very forms of structuring difference according to which both psychic losses and social gains are thought to be culturally and materially distributed? Should we, as Shepherdson claims, discourage individuals from feeling or acting *outside* of the theories which predominate in our understanding of sex/gender or race? Or, like Prosser, do we recognize the ways in which queer or critical race perspectives that invalidate Venus's envious desire for white heterosexual female embodiment—when the successful realization of this very desire might have spared her from the act of transphobic violence that took her life—constitute a theoretical position that "verges on critical perversity"? (1998, 49).[12]

Perversity and pathology are the very terms which have been used to describe the disavowed fantasies of self-constitution that Fanon and Blanchard together explore. In the final analysis, Blanchard's theory of autogynephilia forwards a colorblind and specifically transmisogynistic framework for understanding a desire for trans embodiment that also fails to account for how the very structure of compulsory heterosexuality reproduces those forms of inequality and injustice which continually call forth our envy and outrage. If autogynephilia seems at all compatible with Fanon's anti-racist, anti-colonial message, then it is because his phenomenology of interracial desire is ultimately about an attraction to the "wrong" objects: Fanon appears to offer a description of internalized racism, which is premised on the desirability of the white other, as being inherently paraphilic. Fanon's manipulation of autogynephilic logic additionally portrays cultural imperialism and colonial conquest as psychotic endeavors that seek to deny the magnitude of loss entailed when whiteness is installed as an unquestioned form of social gain.

Despite his pronounced homophobia in *Black Skin*, Fanon's turn to trans embodiment seems to locate a *specifically trans* critique of racism within practices of transformative engagement with white heterosexuality's normative power. Fanon's trans imaginary operates within rather than against notions of psychopathology, drawing subtly upon accounts of gender transition that have contributed to the genealogy of psychosis in the psychiatric and psycho-analytical fields. Given the recent developments in the DSM-V, a trans of color critique is well positioned to reinforce the anti-colonial message Fanon addressed to these fields, which have tended to diagnose psychic injury while ignoring its political causation, and which continue to neglect the fact that medical access is just as important as material support and security for minority subjects, in particular. In Fanon's fleeting moments of attention to gender noncon-formity and variance, we therefore find support for his primary insights: that racism and anti-racist struggle alike can imperil one's mental and physical health; and that it is in the deterritorializing nature of anti-colonial movement building to find oneself aligned with unexpected allies. The publication of the DSM-V has occasioned my particular synthesis of Fanon and Blanchard in this impressionistic commentary on the new paraphilias—one which might cast me as an unwilling apologist of autogynephilia while also leaving me open to the perennial accusation of misappropriating Fanon. On the subject of depathologizing gender nonconformity and variance, however, Fanon invites us to say along with him, "We shall see that another solution is possible. It implies a restructuring of the world" (1967, 82).

Acknowledgements Thanks to Rebecca Garden, William Spurlin, the insightful reviewers for this journal, and the members of the ACLA 2012 seminar on Gender and Sexual Health for their invaluable feedback and encouragement.

Endnotes

[1] Fanon's discussion of the Martinican novelist Mayotte Capécia in the preceding chapter, "The Woman of Color and the White Man," displays this same model of colonized desire, but interestingly does not display its phenomenology: the woman of color never hints at a desire for gender transition.

[2] *Black Skin* seems to have initiated an anti-colonial mode of psychiatric discourse that regards racist injury as synonymous with psychosis. See, for instance, Hickling and Hutchinson (1999). However, this passage still

seems to be in direct conversation with Freud's 1911 study of psychosis centering on the writings of Daniel Paul Schreber, whose religion-tinged delusion is discussed in terms of his identification as a woman (specifically, as God's wife) (Freud 2003).

[3] I use the accepted abbreviation of "trans" to refer to the umbrella category of "transgender," which describes social and cultural phenomena rather than strictly medical designations of identity.

[4] The following regions and countries are represented in the study by Vance, Jr. et al. (2010): Western Europe (Denmark, Finland, Germany, United Kingdom, Netherlands, Spain, Switzerland); East Europe (Russia); North America (Canada, United States); Latin America (Brazil, Chile, Peru); Africa (Nigeria, South Africa, Uganda); Oceania (Australia, New Zealand); and Asia (Kyrgyzstan, Taiwan).

[5] The "transmasculine spectrum" and the "transfeminine spectrum" are terms that attempt to account for the diverse and fluid ways in which gender variant individuals identify and express themselves; they are non-hierarchical and non-teleological models that seek to encompass the full range of trans embodiment (from personal comportment or clothing choice to body modification or gender affirming surgeries) rather than positing an ideal masculine or feminine type (Hansbury 2005).

[6] These internet writings have since been published in Lawrence (2013), which features a foreword by Ray Blanchard.

[7] See also Bailey (2003).

[8] In one of the most direct challenges to Blanchard, Moser (2009) argues that autogynephilic desires can be found in "natal" women, as well, suggesting that femininity functions as an unattainable ideal for all.

[9] See, for instance, Meyer and Richardson (2011).

[10] This rhetoric about the socially-advantageous gender transition is no longer associated with the newly-coined Gender Dysphoria diagnosis in the DSM-V.

[11] The discussion here may seem to invoke the concept of "transableism" or the desire on the part of an able-bodied person to a have a disability or impairment. Comparisons have indeed been made between GID and Body Integrity Identity Disorder (BIID), a condition associated with the elective amputation of one's limbs, but which was never included in the DSM: the DSM-V contains the more general diagnosis of Body Dysmorphic Disorder (BDD). These resonances are too rich to explore fully in this essay, but I will briefly observe that autogynephilia is a paraphilia which entails erotic rather than dysmorphic ideation, e.g., having breasts rather than *not having* a penis, while diagnoses of dysphoria and dysmorphia tend to highlight the role of surgeries in the construction of social identities. An alliance between the disability and trans rights movements is currently being built on the issue of access to appropriate medical care, but transableism remains a controversial term in both communities. See Park (2008) for one side of this controversy.

[12] In a flashpoint of cultural backlash towards Livingston's once-critically-acclaimed project, a New York City audience protested a free Pride-month screening of *Paris* in June 2015, charging the director herself with symbolically and economically appropriating the images and labor of trans and queer people of color. In 1993, over a dozen of the documentary subjects, some of whom were living with HIV, had waged an unsuccessful legal battle for a share of the film's unexpected profits. See Furfaro 2015.

References

American Psychiatric Association. 2000. *Diagnostic and Statistical Manual of Mental Disorders*, 4th ed. https://doi.org/10.1176/appi.books.9780890423349.

———. 2012. "DSM-5 Development: Paraphilias." Accessed 9 March 2012. http://www.dsm5.org/ProposedRevision/Pages/Paraphilias.aspx.

Bailey, J. Michael. 2003. *The Man Who Would be Queen*. Washington, DC: Joseph Henry Press.

Blanchard, Ray. 2005. "Early History of the Concept of Autogynephilia," *Archives of Sexual Behavior* 34:439–446.

———. 2010. "The DSM Diagnostic Criteria for Transvestic Fetishism." *Archives of Sexual Behavior* 39:363–72.

Butler, Judith. 1993. *Bodies That Matter*. New York: Routledge.

———. 1997. *The Psychic Life of Power*. Stanford, CA: Stanford University Press.

Carlson, Shanna T. 2010. "Transgender Subjectivity and the Logic of Sexual Difference." *differences* 21:46–72.

Cheng, Anne. 2001. *Racial Melancholia: Psychoanalysis, Assimilation, and Hidden Grief*. New York: Oxford University Press.

Dean, Tim. 2000. *Beyond Sexuality*. Chicago: University of Chicago Press.

Dreger, Alice. 2008. "The Controversy Surrounding *The Man Who Would Be Queen*." *Archives of Sexual Behavior* 27:366–421.

Eng, David L. and Shinhee Han. 2003. "A Dialogue on Racial Melancholia." In *Loss*, edited by David Eng and David Kazanjian, 343–71. Berkeley, CA: University of California Press.

Fanon, Frantz. 1952. *Peau Noire, Masques Blancs*. Paris: Seuil.

———. 1967. *Black Skin, White Masks*. Translated by Charles Lam Markmann. New York: Grove Press.

———. 2008. *Black Skin, White Masks*. Translated by Richard Philcox. New York: Grove Press.

Freud, Sigmund. (1911) 2003. *The Schreber Case*. New York: Penguin.

———. (1938) 1964. "Findings, Ideas, Problems." In *Standard Edition of the Complete Psychological Works, Volume XXIII*, edited and translated by James Strachey and Anna Freud, 299-300. London, Hogarth Press.

Freund, Kurt and Ray Blanchard. 1993. "Erotic Target Location Errors in Male Gender Dysphorics, Paedophiles, and Fetishists." *The British Journal of Psychiatry* 162:558–63.

Furfaro, Danielle. 2015. "Celebrate Brooklyn fest fails to celebrate trans people of color." *Brooklyn Paper*. Accessed 27 September 2017. https://www.brooklynpaper.com/stories/38/21/dtg-paris-is-burning-controversy-2015-05-22-bk.html.

Hansbury, Griffin. 2005. "The Middle Men: An Introduction to the Transmasculine Identities." *Studies in Gender and Sexuality* 6 (3): 241–264.

Hickling, Frederick W. and Gerard Hutchinson. 1999. "Roast Breadfruit Psychosis: Dsturbed Racial Identification in African-Caribbeans." *Psychiatric Bulletin* 23:132–134.

hooks, bell. 1992. *Black Looks: Race and Representation*. Boston: South End Press.

James, Andrea. 2004. "'Autogynephilia:' A Disputed Diagnosis." *Transsexual Roadmap*. Accessed 30 July 2017. http://www.tsroadmap.com/info/autogynephilia.html.

Lawrence, Anne. 1999. "Men Trapped in Men's Bodies." *Dr. Anne Lawrence on Transsexualism and Sexuality*. Accessed 9 March 2012. http://www.annelawrence.com/1999hbigda2.html.

———. 2007. "Becoming What We Love." *Perspectives in Biology and Medicine* 50:506-520.

———. 2013. *Men Trapped in Men's Bodies: Narratives of Autogynephilic Transsexualism*. New York: Springer.

MacKenzie, Gordene Olga. 1994. *Transgender Nation*. Bowling Green, OH: Bowling Green State University Popular Press.

Meyer, Leisa and Matt Richardson, eds. 2011. "Race and Transgender Studies: A Special Issue." *Feminist Studies* 37 (2).

Moser, Charles. 2009. "Autogynephilia in Women." *Journal of Homosexuality* 56:539-557.

Ngai, Sianne. 2005. *Ugly Feelings*. Cambridge, MA: Harvard University Press.

Park, Pauline. 2008. "The 'Transableism' Phenomenon." Accessed 30 July 2017. http://www.paulinepark.com/2011/01/the-transableism-phenomenon-transsomatechnics-5-2-08/.

Prosser, Jay. 1998. *Second Skins: The Body Narratives of Transsexuality*. New York: Columbia University Press.

Raymond, Janice. 1979. *The Transsexual Empire*. New York: Teachers College Press.

Serano, Julia. 2012. "Trans people still 'disordered' according to latest DSM." Accessed 30 July 2017. http://juliaserano.blogspot.com/2012/12/trans-people-still-disordered-according.html.

Shepherdson, Charles. 2000. *Vital Signs*. New York: Routledge.

Stone, Sandy. 1987. "The 'Empire' Strikes Back: A Posttranssexual Manifesto." Accessed 27 September 2017. https://sandystone.com/empire-strikes-back.pdf.

Stryker, Susan. 2008. *Transgender History*. Berkeley, CA: Seal Press.

Vance, Jr., Stanley R., Peggy T. Cohen-Kettenis, Jack Drescher, Heino F.L. Meyer-Bahlburg, Friedemann Pfällin, and Kenneth J. Zucker. 2010. "Opinions about the DSM Gender Identity Disorder Diagnosis: Results from an International Survey Administered to Organizations Concerned with the Welfare of Transgender People." *International Journal of Transgenderism* 12:1–14.

 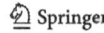

The manufacturer's authorised representative in the EU is Springer
Nature Customer Service Centre GmbH, Europaplatz 3, 69115 Heidelberg,
Germany. If you have any concerns regarding our products, please
contact ProductSafety@springernature.com

Printed and bound by CPI Group (UK) Ltd, Croydon, CR0 4YY
24/04/2026
02096360-0003